Beyond Diet

3 Step Fat Loss

Your Complete Plan to Naturally Lose
Weight and Never Diet Again!

Isabel De Los Rios

Beyond Diet © 2016 by Isabel De Los Rios

First edition published 2007
Second edition published 2008
Third edition published 2009
First hard-copy edition published 2010
Second hard-copy edition published 2010
Third hard-copy edition published 2011
Fourth hard-copy edition published 2011
Fifth hard-copy edition published 2012
Sixth hard-copy edition published 2014
Seventh hard-copy edition published 2015
Eighth hard-copy edition published 2016

Disclaimer

This manual is not intended to provide medical advice or to take the place of medical advice
and treatment from your personal physician. Readers are advised to consult their own doctors
or other qualified health professionals regarding the treatment of medical conditions. The
author shall not be held liable or responsible for any misunderstanding or misuse of the
information contained in this manual or for any loss, damage, or injury caused or alleged to be
caused directly or indirectly by any treatment, action, or application of any food or food source
discussed in this manual. The statements in this book have not be evaluated by the U.S. Food
and Drug Administration. This information is not intended to diagnose, treat, cure, or prevent
any disease.

To request permission for reproduction or inquire about private nutritional
consulting or speaking engagements, contact:

Isabel De Los Rios

Live Smart Solutions

3452 Richville Rd. #1447

Manchester Center, VT 05255

Email: questions@beyonddiet.com

PREFACE

Does the world need another diet book? When I asked myself this question, I knew the answer clearly: No. People don't need another diet book; they need to change their lifestyles. They don't need to be told how and why to go on a diet; they need to learn how to change their eating habits and their thinking for life.

With all the diet books out there, why are so many Americans still overweight and in poor health? Unfortunately, the media bombards us with so much information daily that most people don't know what to believe. I've often heard from clients, "I just don't know what to eat anymore."

With this manual, my goal is to clarify what true nutrition is and which foods you should eat—not only to achieve an ideal weight but also to avoid the conditions that are all too common in this country today, such as high cholesterol, diabetes, and heart disease.

Am I just another nutritionist putting out just another nutrition program? I assure you that I am not. My quest for answers about optimum nutrition began 15 years ago. Since then, I have made it my life's work to study everything I could possibly get my hands on related to nutrition, exercise, and optimum health and weight. This means that I've studied the good and the bad. This manual contains the best information that I've found, culled from some of the most respected doctors and nutritionists who share a similar passion for nutrition.

Like most Americans, I had tried every diet out there and had been unsuccessful in the long term. Only after I recognized and accepted the principles taught in this manual was I able to achieve the optimum weight and health that I enjoy today.

How I nourish my body affects all aspects of my life, as well as my outlook on it. How do I feel when I wake up in the morning? GREAT! How do I feel when I get up in front of a crowd and give a lecture? GREAT! How do I feel when my day doesn't go as planned and things get overwhelming and a bit rough? GREAT!

I know that feeling great has everything to do with how I take care of my body and my health—and you can feel great, too.

Acknowledgements

I thank so many people for making this manual possible:

- God—through whom all things are possible.

- Oscar De Los Rios—whose passion for his work and his life taught me that being passionate about my own work and life is the only way to truly live a happy life.

- Pilar De Los Rios—whose personal struggle with type 2 diabetes and kidney disease taught me more about health and nutrition than any book ever could.

- Every author mentioned in this manual, especially Paul Chek—you have dedicated your lives to studying, researching, and teaching the world what you know is the truth about optimum nutrition. Through your work, I have been able to learn, benefit from, and share this vital information. I am a grateful student forever.

A special thanks to my business partner: Jeff Siegel. His patience and hard work made it possible for this manual to be transformed from an idea to a reality.

CONTENTS

PREFACE 3

ACKNOWLEDGMENTS 5

BEYOND DIET PROGRAM GUIDE................. 10
Step 1 (Days 1-14...................................... 11
Step 2 (Days 15-28).................................... 12
Step 3... 13

THE QUICK START GUIDE........................... 14
The Facts 16
Food Myths, Busted 26
Let's Get Started!...................................... 29
Quick Start FAQs 31

14 DAYS OF SUPERCHARGED MEAL PLANS 35
Introduction.. 36
Frequently Asked Questions 37
Grocery Shopping Guide 39
Day 1... 44
Day 2... 45
Day 3   46
Day 4... 47
Day 5... 48
Day 6... 49
Day 7 - Free Day 50
Day 8... 53

Day 9 54

Day 10 55

Day 11 56

Day 12 57

Day 13 58

Day 14 - Free Day 59

Recipes 60

THE NEXT 14 DAYS OF SUPERCHARGED MEAL PLANS 66

Introduction 67

Grocery Shopping Guide 68

Day 1 73

Day 2 74

Day 3 75

Day 4 76

Day 5 77

Day 6 78

Day 7 - Free Day 79

Day 8 81

Day 9 82

Day 10 83

Day 11 84

Day 12 85

Day 13 86

Day 14 - Free Day 87

Recipes 88

BEYOND DIET MANUAL 102

1: A Program for Success 103
2: Three Steps to Weight Loss 107
3: Metabolism Types.................................. 113
4: Calories 121
5: Daily Meal Planning 129
6: Organic Food 135
7: Fats 142
8: Dairy 151
9: Soy 158
10: Grains 162
11: Salt... 172
12: Water... 176
13: Sweeteners 180
14: Superfoods 190
15: Alcohol 199
16: Supplements 202
17: Vegetarians....................................... 206
18: Recipe Guide Overview 208

THE SHOPPING GUIDE 211

Getting Started....................................... 212
Staple Foods Shopping List........................ 213
Understanding The Universal Layout............. 219
Selecting Quality Foods............................. 222
Healthy Condiments 234
Healthy Snacks....................................... 242
Organic on the Cheap............................... 245

ADVANCED MEAL PLANNING 255

Getting Started...256
Meal Planning Tools 257
Planning Your Meals..261
Adding Food and Recipes..................................263
Meal Planning Next Steps..................................267

METABOLISM TYPE TEST 268

Questions..269
Scoring...273

GUIDES & CHARTS 274

Cooking with Fats 275
Allowable Servings Guide 277
Food Choices 280
Ideal Food Ratios for Each Metabolism Type 290
Glycemic Index Chart 291
Good, Better, Best..293

SO...JUST WHO IS ISABEL DE LOS RIOS?....298

REFERENCES... 300

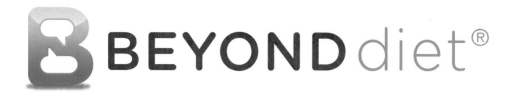

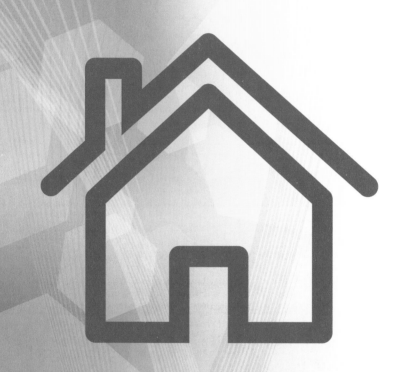

PROGRAM GUIDE

Isabel De Los Rios

This Program Guide will show you the best and easiest way to get started with Beyond Diet. These three steps simplify all of the great information you get inside Beyond Diet into one easy how-to... just for you!

I want you to commit to giving this program 4 weeks. You will see a difference in less than 7 days, and after the first 2 weeks, you'll be feeling great. But after 4 weeks you will know which foods to eat to lose weight, and you'll be feeling amazing!

For the best results, it is highly recommended that you follow the steps as outlined below.

Step 1 (Days 1-14)

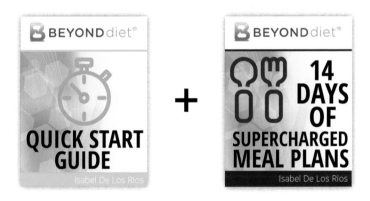

Read the Quick Start Guide and follow the 14 Days of Supercharged Meal Plans.

The Quick Start Guide is the first step to success – this is where you will learn the basics of the Beyond Diet program.

The 14 Days of Supercharged Meal Plans are super simple, and they will be very effective at jump starting your weight loss.

Once you have read the Quick Start Guide and completed

the 14 Days of Supercharged Meal Plans, it's time to have you understand the underlying principles of the Beyond Diet program so you can truly enjoy the transition to this new, healthy eating lifestyle.

Step 2 (Days 15-28)

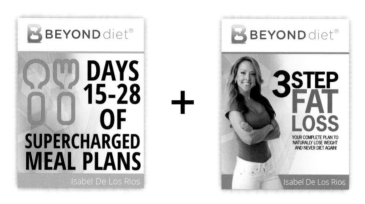

Step 2 is to follow the Supercharged Meal Plans, Days 15-28 while you read the Beyond Diet Manual. The next 14 days of Supercharged Meal Plans will help you continue to lose weight with delicious, fat-burning recipes.

The Beyond Diet Manual will walk you through all the tools and information you need to know to keep losing fat and achieve the body you've always wanted.

Step 3

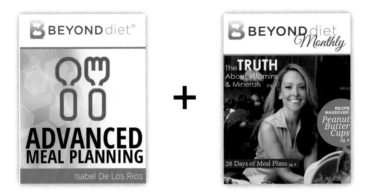

Now that you have a good understanding of the principles of Beyond Diet – and have already started seeing the results of the program – you can start creating your own meal plans. Or start using BD Monthly, which gives you 28 days of fresh, fat-burning meal plans every month.

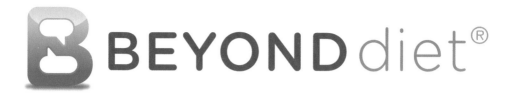

BEYOND diet®

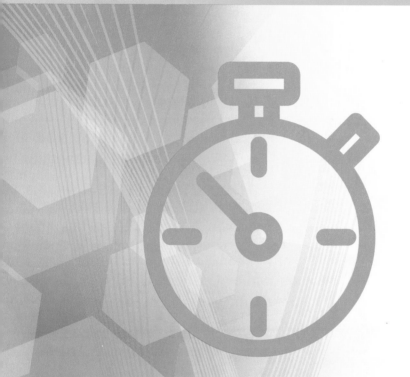

QUICK START
GUIDE

Isabel De Los Rios

Congratulations on your decision to live a healthier life. I am so excited to be on this wonderful journey alongside you.

Now that you have this program, you will see all the wonderful information Beyond Diet has to offer. In order to ensure your success, I highly recommend you follow the steps to following this program as I have outlined for you (if you are reading this Quick Start Guide first, you are in the right place).

Reading this Quick Start Guide is your first step to success. I have made each topic easy to read and simple to understand. Don't worry. We will go into each topic in more depth later in the program, but right now all you need to do is read through the Quick Start Guide and then I will tell you where to go next. Sound like a plan?

You will see that there are many eye opening topics and principles presented in this program. They are the exact principles that have helped thousands of people lose weight and make a permanent change in their lives.

As with any new change in your life, you may have some questions or just need a little extra help along the way. That is why we have created the Beyond Diet community.

Are you ready to get started? Let's jump right in!

A journey of a thousand miles begins with a single step. Start now!

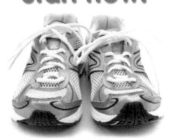

The Facts

Get ready to feel awesome!

Below are the simple facts you need to know in order to successfully begin the first set of Beyond Diet Meal Plans. Just knowing these facts will arm you with a wealth of knowledge to be successful in the first few weeks. Each topic will be covered in more depth later in the program, but for now, this is the perfect place to start.

1. Set up your mind for success.

The first principle we're going to cover has nothing to do with food at all, but has everything to do with your health and your success on this program. What many people don't realize is that the thoughts they think each day can affect their weight loss dramatically.

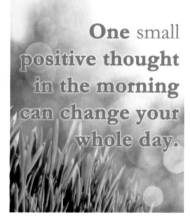

Consider this...

Let's say Sally and Joe both start the Beyond Diet program on the same day. Sally goes into the program with the mind set, "This is going to be great. I can already see my new body coming!" Joe, on the other hand, starts the program with the completely opposite mind set, "Oh what's the use? I've tried to lose weight so many other times. I guess I'll just see if I fail at this too."

If you had to guess, which person do you think has a greater chance of reaching their weight loss goals? Yup, Sally. Because she started off in the right mind set.

I'm asking you to do the same. I'm asking you to start this program with an open mind and to know that you too can be as successful as thousands of other people who have lost weight using these methods.

Spend some time today thinking and writing down exactly what you want for your health, your weight, and your life. See yourself in the healthy, beautiful body you've always dreamed about and believe it is possible for you.

(If you haven't done so already, please be sure to add your visualization to your profile on BeyondDiet.com. I'm excited to read it!).

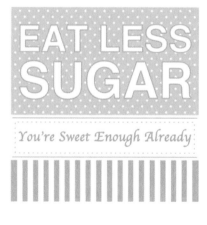

2. Let's kick sugar once and for all!

It is no longer a secret or even a shock to most people that refined sugar causes weight gain and is one of the leading causes of obesity in the world. Sugar is also extremely addictive (causing feelings of highs and lows in the body similar to most drugs). And the negative side effects are just as bad as drugs, if not worse.

Americans, truly, don't realize how much sugar they are consuming in one day. Most soft drinks, juices and even some "health" drinks have anywhere between 5-10 teaspoons [25-50 mL] of sugar in each 8 oz [236 mL] serving. Can you imagine putting 8 oz [236 mL] of water in a cup, adding 10 teaspoons [50 mL] of white sugar, and then drinking it? Well this is exactly what you are doing when you drink any kind of soft drink, juice and most other drinks on the market today.

And it's not just drinks that are loaded with sugar. Most cereals and packaged foods have sugar (or some form of sugar) listed as the first or second ingredient (which means it is the ingredient in the highest quantity). The following words on a nutritional label mean "sugar" and should probably be avoided:

Corn Sweetener, Corn Syrup, or Corn Syrup Solids, Dehydrated Cane Juice, Dextrin, Dextrose, Fructose, Fruit Juice Concentrate, Glucose, High Fructose Corn Syrup, Lactose, Maltodextrin, Malt Syrup, Maltose, Raw Sugar, Rice Syrup, Saccharose, Sucrose, Syrup, Treacle, Turbinado Sugar, Xylose

Fortunately for those looking for a lean, defined body, once you stop eating sugar, your addiction will quickly disappear. People who are "on" sugar crave it all the time. People who are "off" sugar don't even miss it. Weaning yourself off sugar and sugar containing products will cause a drastic and immediate change in your weight. The first few days may be a bit of a "detox" (just like a drug), but these symptoms quickly disappear (and so do the pounds!).

3. Artificial Sweeteners are NOT a good replacement to sugar.

Many times when people decide to give up sugar, they quickly resort to artificial sweeteners. Artificial sweeteners are definitely not the answer! Sorbitol, saccharin, aspartame and sucralose are actually worse for you than sugar itself. All of these artificial sweeteners have been linked to cancer, tumors, and obesity. Yes, artificial sweeteners cause weight gain by disrupting your body's natural hormones. Studies have shown that when people give up their daily "Diet Drink" (filled with aspartame) they quickly lose up to 10 pounds [4.5 kilos] just by eliminating the consumption of this toxic sweetener.

So it is equally important to eliminate any food that contains the above mentioned sweeteners as it is to eliminate sugar from your daily intake.

Most people's next question is then, "Well what is left if I want something sweet?" A great alternative to sugar and artificial sweeteners is the supplement STEVIA. Stevia is a naturally sweet plant native to Paraguay that is 30 times sweeter than sugar in its unprocessed form. With hundreds of studies showing stevia is a safe alternative, it's the next big thing. No wonder. It's all-natural, contains zero calories, and has a zero glycemic index. Stevia leaves are 250-400 times sweeter than sugar and perfect for helping anyone wean themselves away from refined white sugar and artificial sweeteners. Stevia products are great for beverages, soft foods, and baking. Stevia products are available in most local natural foods and health food stores. In grocery stores, Stevia products are typically found in the health food aisle with other supplements.

4. Let's go back to eating "real food."

Have you noticed how much fatter Americans have gotten since more "weight loss" and "diet" foods have been put out on

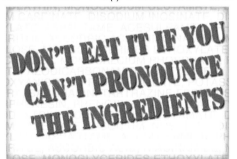

the market? Well, I assure you it's no coincidence. Processed foods can truly be considered "Non Foods" since they resemble more of a science experiment than they do real food.

To make differentiating between healthy natural food vs. non-foods easy, just stay away from anything that contains ingredients on a label that you can't pronounce. If the ingredients list to your favorite cereal is more complicated than your college organic chemistry final, chances are you should stay away from it at all costs. These chemicals are all toxins to your body (just as artificial sweeteners are) and your liver becomes extremely overwhelmed trying to rid your body of these harmful toxins. Why is this important in your efforts to lose fat? Well, the other job of your liver is to burn body fat and if it is too busy ridding you of toxic overload, it has no time (or energy) to get rid of your unwanted fat.

5. Eat the "right carbs" for optimal health and fat loss.

I do agree that reducing the amount of carbohydrates in your meal plans will help you lose weight and lean down. But you must reduce the bad and increase the good. Eating fibrous carbohydrates like fruits and vegetables actually turns your body into a fat burning machine. Eating starchy carbs like rice and potatoes after a workout will also help you develop the lean, muscular physique most men and women are looking for. It is the processed and refined wheat and grains that are causing everyone to feel bloated and have a difficult time losing weight.

Don't fall into the "no carb" trap. Learn the right carb approach to look great and feel great.

6. Fire up your metabolism by eating regularly. (Don't eat like a sumo wrestler!)

Sumo wrestlers make a concerted effort to get fat for their sport. So if your number one goal was to GET FAT this is exactly what you could do:

1. Skip breakfast and eat very little all day long.

2. Eat the bulk of your caloric intake in a large heavy meal, filled with complex carbohydrates in the evening.

3. Go to bed after eating this heavy meal.

That's it. This strategy has been working for sumo wrestlers for years. And you know who else it is working for? The 130 million Americans who are overweight or obese.

You must develop the habit of eating frequent meals all day 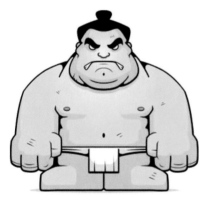 long to develop the kind of warp speed metabolism that is going to allow you to get lean and stay lean (no sense in getting there without being able to maintain it right?) Eat 4-6 well portioned meals each day and you will see your body burn fat faster than you can say "sumo wrestler."

7. Water, it does a body good.

If you often feel like you are starving all day no matter how much food you've consumed, chances are you may be severely dehydrated. Many people actually mistake dehydration for hunger and eat tons more calories than they actually need when all they really needed to do was drink some water!

It would be impossible to pick up any diet or weight loss book without it saying somewhere "drink 8-10 cups of water each day." Even if all health and nutrition gurus don't agree on all the same principles, they do all agree on one: water is the magic potion to ensure weight loss. When you consider that water helps the body metabolize stored fat, rid the body of waste (as in unwanted fats and toxins), and is a natural diuretic and a natural laxative, no wonder it is an absolute MUST when fat loss is your goal. Drink a minimum of 1/2 of your body weight in ounces of filtered water each day to ensure that your body rids itself of the unwanted fat you are aiming to lose.

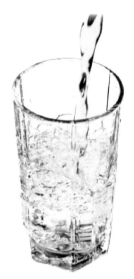

8. Throw out all those deceiving "health foods."

Yes, you have been scammed. You and approximately hundreds of thousands of other people who have purchased pre-packaged "health" foods. There are many health foods on the market today that are causing people to gain weight, as well as making it near impossible for them to lose weight. Have you ever purchased the foods that someone claimed to be "guaranteed to make you lose weight" only to see the scale go up instead of down? Frustrated dieters all over the world can't figure out why their new weight loss shake is not working like the commercial suggested. Well, one of the nasty culprits causing millions of people to pack on the pounds is hydrogenated oil. There are thousands of health foods that contain this toxic oil. Weight Watchers and Lean Cuisine meals and bars almost all contain hydrogenated oil (and they are supposed to be good for you?). Even some energy sports bars and shakes are loaded up with hydrogenated oils and many other toxic preservatives.

Another nasty culprit is processed soy. This is always a shock to most people (especially die-hard vegetarians) who have been falsely led to believe that soy is actually good for you. Well if you lived in Asia you would quickly see that most Asians eat soy in small quantities in the form of old fashioned fermented soy (such as miso, tempeh, natto, shoyu, and tamari) not the processed, toxic soy that is used in so many vegetarian type products and weight loss products on the market today. The worst of today's soy protein products are soy protein isolate, soy protein concentrate, texturized vegetable protein and hydrolyzed vegetable protein. These ingredients are found in everything from shake powders, energy bars and veggie burgers to canned tuna. The worst soy oil products are margarines and shortenings made from partially hydrogenated soybean oil containing dangerous trans fatty acids. So avoid these forms of toxic soy at all costs. Not only will you be saving yourself from a myriad of health problems (like decreased thyroid function and hormone disruption) you will also see a dramatic loss in unwanted body fat.

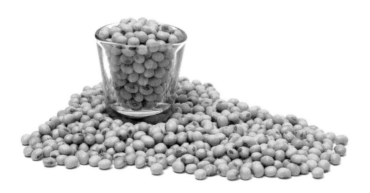

9. Learn to love fat... I mean the *right kind* of fat.

While some thought Atkins was the best thing since sliced bread, others thought that fat was the root of all evil. This is only partially true, and the complete elimination of all fats from your diet is a BIG mistake. Yes, you should eliminate 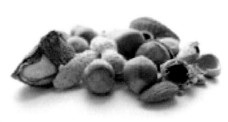 unhealthy fats like hydrogenated oils (sorry, that means no French fries or doughnuts). But the healthy fats found in wild fish and nuts are absolutely necessary for your body to function at optimum. These fats, called Omega-3 essential fatty acids, are actually so critical to your body's functioning, that it is very difficult to experience any weight loss without including them in your meal plan.

Where do you find these Omega-3s? You find them in salmon, walnuts, chia seeds, and organic eggs. Make these foods an integral part of your eating regimen and you will see some great results in your weight loss efforts.

A high quality Omega-3 supplement also ensures you get your daily dose, works wonders for your body, and helps to burn off unwanted fat. This is my personal favorite and the one I take every day: http://go.beyonddiet.com/Omega3.

10. Build your body and stop hunger by eating protein.

Protein is not just for bodybuilders. It's for every person who wants to achieve a lean, slender and toned physique. (Did I just describe every person on the planet?) Protein not only fuels your muscles, it also helps stabilize your blood sugar and prevents hunger. So you get the benefit of lean, toned muscles and a way to NOT be hungry. Sounds like a win, win to me. Unfortunately, most people go the entire day without eating any protein at all. It's no wonder these are the same people that complain of a flabby body, fatigue, and hunger pangs that just won't go away. Include a source of healthy protein into each meal (that includes snacks). Wonderful sources of protein are grass fed meats, free range poultry, organic eggs, wild fish, and organic raw nuts.

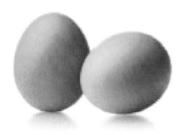

Food Myths, Busted

1. Cola is worse than you think.

Soda is absolutely toxic for your body. Just look at the ingredients label of a can of soda. One of the first two ingredients is likely high fructose corn syrup, an ingredient that should be avoided at all costs. While most people are aware of the dangers of drinking regular soda, many people falsely believe that "diet" soda is in some way a good thing for losing body fat when, in fact, there is absolutely nothing healthy about drinking diet soda. Diet soda tricks your sweet tooth into thinking you're getting something for nothing, which can actually lead to overeating. Worse yet, drinking soda is associated with obesity, diabetes, heart disease, liver damage, high blood pressure, osteoporosis, even some cancers.

2. Did you know salt is good for you?

You don't need to cut salt out completely, but you do need to change the type of salt you use. Salt has such a bad reputation because 99% of the world's salt research has been done on commercial table salt.

Instead of refined table salt, use unrefined sea salt or Himalayan rock salt. These salts are extremely healthy and have the exact opposite effect of refined salt. They provide sodium chloride in a form that the body needs to function and offer the perfect balance of minerals, nutrients, and sodium chloride that the body needs for optimum health.

3. Eating the right kind of bread is critical to weight loss success.

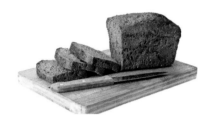

Bread is a staple of the American diet. Unfortunately, most of us eat the absolute worst kind of bread: the kind made from refined grains. White bread is stripped of essential vitamins and nutrients during processing, and the whole wheat bread the American public has been led to believe is healthy contains processed wheat, which is deficient in nutrients. If you are not willing to forgo eating bread altogether, I suggest you look into stocking your fridge with sprouted whole grain (SWG) bread.

4. Cook with butter or coconut oil.

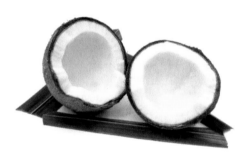

Fake butters are made from unhealthy, unnatural ingredients which are perceived as toxins in the body. As I've mentioned, it is your liver's job to filter these unnatural ingredients out of your bloodstream. The more work your liver as to do, the harder it is to maintain a healthy weight. Replace those fake butters with raw, organic butter. This is actually one of the healthiest whole foods you can include in your diet.

Another great oil to incorporate into your eating plan every day is unrefined coconut oil. Besides the fact that it tastes amazing, it has been called a "miracle" food by physicians and health professionals for its ability to speed up the metabolism and help the body burn off unwanted fat.

5. No more canola oil.

When answering the question "is canola oil bad for you?" most people have focused on the fact that canola oil was, originally, a derivative of rapeseed oil. Rapeseed oil, beyond having the kind of name that makes you want to stay away, contains high levels of erucic acid, which is associated with heart disease. In the past several decades, farmers and researchers selectively bred rapeseed in order to lower the amount of erucic acid found in the oils.

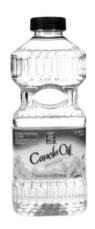

But even if you don't have to worry that you're cooking your heart healthy meals in an oil that may cause heart disease, the larger – and unavoidable – problem with canola oil cannot be ignored.

Most seeds used to make canola oil in the United States are genetically modified. Canola seeds are planted in massive fields, and nearly 80% of those seeds have been genetically modified so farmers can spray their fields with weed killers without also killing the crops. So using canola oil means putting something in your body that has been modified to withstand industrial pesticides.

Canola oil is heavily processed. After being extracted from the seeds, canola oil is chemically refined, bleached with organic acids, and deodorized, so the oil you use to cook will neither look nor smell as it does naturally.

Polyunsaturated fats oxidize under high heat. Oxidization can occur either during processing or cooking. The oxidization of polyunsaturated fats releases free radicals into the body, increasing your risk for many diseases, including cancer.

Let's Get Started!

Wow! Did you learn a lot? I hope you did. Because it is my #1 goal to give you all of the information you need to not only drop your unwanted fat for good, but also make you feel great every single day.

Right around this point is where people ask me, "Isabel, now what do you want me to do with all of this information?"

Lucky for you, I have figured out a way to make this as easy for you as possible (not to mention showing you incredible results in the least amount of time).

I have created for you very easy-to-follow meal plans that you will be using for the next 14 days. These meal plans will help you to apply the principles you just learned, without having to figure any of this out yourself. I've done all the work for you.

Sound good?

So your next step is to open up the 14 Day Meal Plans and all the instructions you need are there.

But before you go… I have a few more items to let you know about:

Because I know any lifestyle change can bring up a lot of questions, we have set up the Beyond Diet website so you always have a place to get all of your questions answered and to share your successes along the way. I want you to know…

We are here for you! Please remember that. I do not want you to ever feel like you are in this alone. That is why we have created the ASK and SHARE sections in Beyond Diet.

Please ASK Us

If you have a specific question about following the meal plans or any of the information you have just read, please ask it in the ASK section (you can find the ASK section on the homepage of the members area). You will see that you are first given the option to search for an answer to your question (your specific question may have already been answered on the site). If you do not see the answer, click to ask a new question. Our coaches and other Beyond Diet members will answer any question you might have!

Please SHARE With Us

If you would like to share any detail about your life or your health journey, please share it with our loving community in the SHARE section (you can also find the SHARE section on the home page of your members area). You will see what a true family we are in Beyond Diet and how encouraging and helpful everyone is. We love to hear your successes as well as any challenges that may come up along the way. Please post those in the SHARE section. I look forward to reading them!

Quick Start FAQs

Here are the answers to a whole bunch of questions you should know right now:

When should I read the manual?

Many people get very excited when they see all of the great information Beyond Diet has to offer. I am equally as excited for you to learn more and more about how to keep your body lean, toned and super healthy.

But...

I highly recommend you start reading the Beyond Diet Manual AFTER you have completed the 14 Day Meal Plans. Why would I make that suggestion? Because I want your #1 focus right now to be following the first 2 weeks of meal plans in the best way possible.

What I have seen happen in the past is that people start to read the manual as they are following the 14 Day Meal Plans and they start to become overwhelmed by all of the information they have in front of them. I assure you, if you follow the plan I have outlined for you, in the order I have given, that is the best way I can guarantee your success.

When should I start taking my Daily Energy greens drink?

You can start benefiting from all the healthy vitamins, minerals, and superfoods in Daily Energy right away! The best time to drink Daily Energy is in the morning, right before your breakfast. This will give you tons of energy all day long and get your day started in the perfect way.

If you have not purchased Daily Energy yet, you can do so here:

http://go.beyonddiet.com/DailyEnergy

Should I purchase the Omega-3 supplement you mentioned earlier?

I would absolutely love it if every person beginning this program also started taking a high quality Omega-3 supplement shortly after beginning the meal plans. (NOTE: You do not need to wait to get your Omega-3 supplement to get started on the 14 Day Meal Plans.)

Many people, and this may include you, beginning a healthy eating plan are extremely deficient in Omega-3s and it can affect your ability to burn off unwanted fat. Incorporating an Omega-3 supplement into your diet can greatly enhance and accelerate your weight loss results.

Get my favorite Omega-3 supplement here: http://go.beyonddiet.com/Omega3

When can I use all the great recipes on the website?

You are soon going to see how wonderful this way of eating really is and I know you're going to be excited to try new recipes in the kitchen. Hang tight! That will come very soon. We will start using all of the amazing recipes inside the Beyond Diet site once you have completed these 2 weeks.

Right now our goal is to keep this as simple and as easy to follow to ensure your success. Following the program as I have outlined it for you will guarantee the best results.

When can I start using the Success Journal?

You will start using the Success Journal after these first 2 weeks of plans. The Success Journal is a wonderful tool that you are going to love, but I will be teaching you how to use it properly when we get into the Beyond Diet program manual.

When should I start exercising?

You can start exercising right away or continue on your current exercise program. If you are not currently involved in some form of exercise program, you can begin by just incorporating some simple walking into your daily routine.

I also recommend participating in activities outside or with your children, as those forms of exercise are the most fun!

When can I start using the other components I purchased (ex: recipe books, smart coaching, additional meal plans and exercise programs)?

All of these components are great and you will find that they are really going to help you be successful on the Beyond Diet program. But we are going to use those when we get into the main manual.

I know you may be anxious to dive into all of your great stuff, but please be patient, it will all come together soon and trying to do too much all at once can be detrimental to your success.

The only exception to this rule is with any of the exercise programs you have purchased. If you have already been cleared by your physician to start exercising, you can begin these programs right away.

What if I can't find the foods on the meal plans?

We give you a full shopping list to use when shopping for foods you need to follow these meal plans. Most of the foods can be found at your local grocery store, health food store, or farmer's market. Some foods may be better purchased online.

If you have any questions about sourcing a specific food, please post about it in the DISCUSS section.

What if I follow the 14 Day Meal Plans for a few days and don't see any results?

It is very unlikely that this will happen, as most people will already feel a difference within the first few days. Please do not use the scale as your guide. Use how you feel and how your clothes are fitting as a better indicator of whether or not the meal plans are working.

It is extremely important you follow the meal plans for the entire 2 weeks (unless you are medically unable to continue). Some people see more results in the second week than in the first.

I can assure you that if you stick to the program as it is written, it will work for you!

What if I have a question that isn't answered above?

We are always available to help. You can ask your question in the ASK or DISCUSS sections of the site and someone will give you an answer as quickly as possible.

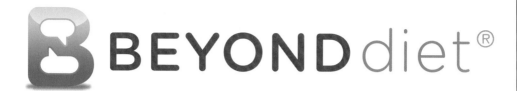

14 DAYS OF

SUPERCHARGED
MEAL PLANS

Isabel De Los Rios

Introduction

I'm so excited for you to get started on these meal plans. In just a few days from now, you will already see a big difference in how you look and how you feel!

These meal plans were created to help you easily implement all of the information you learned in the Quick Start Guide.

Please be sure to read all of the instructions and take a look through the Shopping Guides and Meal Plans before beginning the 14 Days of Supercharged Meal Plans.

How to Use These Meal Plans

There are 12 meal plans for you to follow. You will follow the meal plans for 6 days and then give yourself a "free day" (more info on that later) on Day 7. You will then follow the meal plans for another 6 days and give yourself another "free day" on Day 14.

Please take some time now to look through the Shopping Guide and the Meal Plans and some general questions I have answered for you on the next page.

Frequently Asked Questions

What if there is a meal or food I don't like?

I understand that each of us has different tastes and that some of these meals may taste great to you while some may not appeal to you at all. You can easily adjust your meals for the day by choosing the breakfasts you like, the snack you like... etc...and mix and match them to create your own meal plans. Each meal is interchangeable. Just don't exchange a breakfast with a lunch or a lunch with a dinner. You can only exchange the same type of meal (breakfast with breakfast, lunch with lunch).

Do I need to modify these meal plans based on my weight?

The meal plans are roughly based on a 1600 calorie meal plan. I have found that 1600 calories of the right food combinations is sufficient to keep most people from being hungry while simultaneously quickly burning off a lot of body fat.

If you have been a dieter for a long time and 1600 sounds a bit high to you, I assure you it's not. Restricting calories to low levels can be damaging to your metabolism and make your body hold on to fat instead of burning it off. Also, the foods that I have chosen in these meal plans are foods that will naturally stimulate fat burning in your body.

If you feel like you need more food, and are hungry while following these plans, you can begin by increasing the protein servings by 1 ounce at a time. For example, if lunch calls for 4 oz salmon, increase it to 5 or 6 if necessary.

Remember, also, that these meal plans are to be followed for 2 weeks. You will then be creating new meal plans for yourself that are specific to your own personal needs. (We'll get to that later in the Main Manual.)

What can I drink while following these meal plans?

1. Water - 1/2 of your body weight in ounces of water each day (e.g. if you weigh 150 pounds, then 75 ounces of water throughout the course of each day)

2. Green Tea - (careful with the caffeine content) sweetened with stevia

3. Coffee - (1 cup maximum) sweetened with stevia (no milk or creamer)

How much weight should I expect to lose with these meal plans?

You can expect to lose anywhere between 5-10 pounds in these first 2 weeks...some people may lose more, some people may lose less. Please do not focus so much on the number on the scale, but focus more on how you feel, how your clothes are fitting and the wonderful habits you are changing in these first 2 weeks.

Grocery Shopping Guide

Week 1 – Days 1 through 6

(*Some products purchased during week 1 will be left over to use for week 2)

Produce	Amount	Notes
Apples (Green)	6	Small
Avocado	2-3	
Banana	3 1/2	
Bay Leaf	1	
Bell Peppers	3	Any color - Make sure one is red.
Berries	1 1/2 cups	Any berries - strawberries, blueberries, raspberries, blackberries.
Broccoli	4 cups	
Carrots	6-8	Medium
Cauliflower	1 cup	
Celery	3-4 stalks	
Cherry Tomatoes	2-3 cups	
Cucumbers	2	
Garlic	1 head	
Greens (Mixed)	5 cups	Romaine, Arugula, Red Leaf, or Bibb Lettuce
Green Beans	1 cup	
Onions	2	
Plum Tomatoes	2 cups	
Spaghetti Squash	1	Small
Spinach	6 cups	

Produce (cont.)	Amount	Notes
Sweet Potato	1	
Tomatoes	6	
Zucchini	3	
Meat & Seafood	**Amount**	**Notes**
Bacon	6 slices	Nitrate-Free, Uncured, Pork or Turkey
Ground Buffalo	1 pound	Can substitute ground beef
Chicken Breast	8 ounces	Free-Range
Chicken Thighs	18 ounces	Free-Range
Halibut	10 ounces	
Salmon	4 ounces	
Sausage	3 ounces	Chicken, Turkey, or Pork
Ground Turkey	1 1/2 pounds	Free-Range
Sliced Turkey	4 ounces	Nitrate-Free
Eggs & Dairy	**Amount**	**Notes**
Eggs	4	Cage-Free, Organic
Nuts & Seeds	**Amount**	**Notes**
Raw Almonds	2 ounces	
Raw Macadamia Nuts	1 ounce	
Raw Nut Butter	1 jar	Almond Butter, Walnut Butter, or Cashew Butter
Raw Pumpkin Seeds	1 ounce	
Raw Walnuts	1 ounce	
Miscellaneous	**Amount**	**Notes**
Coconut Oil	1 jar	
Extra Virgin Olive Oil	1 bottle	

Miscellaneous (cont.)	Amount	Notes
Raw/Organic Butter	1 stick	
Apple Cider Vinegar	1 bottle	
Soy Sauce	1 bottle	Wheat-Free
Chicken Stock/Broth	1 cup	
Dijon Mustard	1 jar	
Daily Energy	1	http://go.beyonddiet.com/DailyEnergy
Omega-3 Supplement	1	http://go.beyonddiet.com/Omega3
Parmesan Cheese	1	
Seasonings	**Amount**	**Notes**
Basil (Fresh)	1	
Black Pepper	1	
Cayenne Pepper	1	
Chili Powder	1	
Ground Cumin	1	
Garlic Powder	1	
Oregano (Dried)	1	
Paprika	1	
Parsley (Dried & Fresh)	1 each	
Unrefined Sea Salt	1	http://go.beyonddiet.com/AztecSeaSalt
Thyme (Dried)	1	

Week 2 – Days 8 through 13

Produce	Amount	Notes
Apples (Green)	7	
Avocado	2	
Bananas	3	
Bay Leaf	1	
Bell Peppers	3	Any color - Make sure one is red.
Berries	1 cup	Any berries - strawberries, blueberries, raspberries, blackberries.
Broccoli	4 cups	
Carrots	6-8	Medium
Cauliflower	2 cups	
Celery	2-3 stalks	
Cherry Tomatoes	2-3 cups	
Cucumbers	2	
Garlic	1 head	
Greens (Mixed)	5 cups	Romaine, Arugula, Red Leaf, or Bibb Lettuce
Green Beans	1 cup	
Onions	2	
Plum Tomatoes	2 cups	
Romaine Lettuce	1 cup	
Spaghetti Squash	1	Small
Spinach	5 cups	
Tomatoes	7	
Zucchini	3	

Meat & Seafood	Amount	Notes
Bacon	6 slices	Nitrate-Free, Uncured, Pork or Turkey
Ground Buffalo	1 pound	Can substitute ground beef
Chicken Breast	9 ounces	Free-Range
Chicken Thighs	11 ounces	Free-Range
Halibut	10 ounces	
Salmon	8 ounces	
Sausage	3 ounces	Chicken, Turkey, or Pork
Ground Turkey	1 1/2 pounds	Free-Range
Sliced Turkey	8 ounces	Nitrate-Free
Eggs & Dairy	**Amount**	**Notes**
Eggs	6	Cage-Free, Organic
Nuts & Seeds	**Amount**	**Notes**
Raw Almonds	2 ounces	
Raw Macadamia Nuts	1 ounce	
Raw Pumpkin Seeds	1 ounce	
Raw Walnuts	1 ounce	

Day 1

Food	Serving	Notes
Breakfast		
Cage-Free, Organic Eggs	2 eggs	Suggested: Cook the spinach using coconut oil and then add in the eggs (lightly beaten) to make a spinach omelet. Eat it over the sliced tomato.
Fresh Spinach	1 cup	
Fresh Tomatoes	1 cup	
Unrefined Virgin Coconut Oil	2 tsp	
Daily Energy Greens Drink	1 serving	
Morning Snack		
Raw Almonds	1 oz	
Fresh Banana	1/2 banana	
Lunch		
Fresh Wild Caught Salmon	4 oz	Suggested: Broil the salmon with salt and pepper. Can do this the night before to have it ready for lunch. Eat it cold over the salad.
Super Simple Side Salad	1 salad	
Isabel's Famous Salad Dressing	1-2 Tbsp	
Granny Smith Apple	1 apple	
Afternoon Snack		
Chicken Breast	4 oz	Suggested: Bake the sweet potato in the oven for 45 minutes. Steam the broccoli.
Organic Broccoli	1 cup	
Organic Sweet Potato	1/2 cup	
Dinner		
Turkey Chili	1 serving	This Turkey Chili recipe makes 4 servings. Eat 1 serving for dinner and 1 serving for lunch tomorrow. The remaining 2 servings can be shared with family or saved for next week.

Day 2

Food	Serving	Notes
Breakfast		
Sausage (chicken, turkey, or pork)	3 oz	Suggested: Cut up the onions and pepper and cook in coconut oil. Then add in sausage.
Bell Pepper (any color)	1/2 cup	
Onion (any type)	1/2 cup	
Unrefined Virgin Coconut Oil	2 tsp	
Daily Energy Greens Drink	1 serving	
Morning Snack		
Granny Smith Apple	1 apple	
Raw Almonds	1 oz	
Lunch		
Turkey Chili	1 serving	Lunch will be leftovers from last night's dinner
Afternoon Snack		
Organic Carrots	1 cup	
Raw Nut Butter	2 Tbsp	
Dinner		
Organic, Free-Range Chicken Thigh	4 oz	
Garlic Green Beans	1 serving	
Cucumber and Tomato Salad	1 serving	
Isabel's Famous Salad Dressing	1-2 Tbsp	

Day 3

Food	Serving	Notes
Breakfast		
Nitrate-Free Organic Bacon	3 oz	
Cage-Free Organic Egg	1 egg	
Fresh Tomatoes	1 cup	
Daily Energy Greens Drink	1 serving	
Morning Snack		
Raw Macadamia Nuts	1/2 oz	
Fresh Mixed Berries	1/2 cup	
Lunch		
Organic, Free-Range Chicken Thigh	4 oz	Suggested: Cut up the chicken and avocado and add them to the salad.
Organic Avocado	2 oz	
Super Simple Side Salad	1 salad	
Isabel's Famous Salad Dressing	1-2 Tbsp	
Granny Smith Apple	1 apple	
Afternoon Snack		
Fresh Banana	1 banana	
Raw Nut Butter	2 Tbsp	
Dinner		
Turkey Burgers	1 serving	Suggested: Cut up the peppers and onions and saute them in coconut oil. The Turkey Burger recipe makes 2 burgers - eat 1 for dinner and save the other for tomorrow's lunch.
Sauteed Spinach	1 serving	
Bell Pepper (any color)	1/2 cup	
Onion (any type)	1/2 onion	
Unrefined Virgin Coconut Oil	1 tsp	

Day 4

Food	Serving	Notes
Breakfast		
Organic, Free-Range Chicken Thigh	3 oz	Suggested: Cut up the chicken and avocado and serve them over steamed cauliflower.
Organic Avocado	1 oz	
Organic Cauliflower	1 cup	
Daily Energy Greens Drink	1 serving	
Morning Snack		
Organic Carrot	1 cup	
Raw Nut Butter	2 Tbsp	
Lunch		
Turkey Burgers	1 serving	
Celery and Carrots	1 cup	
Granny Smith Apple	1 apple	
Afternoon Snack		
Sliced Turkey	4 oz	
Organic Cucumber	1 cup	
Fresh Tomatoes	1 cup	
Dinner		
Organic, Free-Range Chicken Thigh	4 oz	
Organic Broccoli	1 cup	
Super Simple Side Salad	1 salad	
Isabel's Famous Salad Dressing	1-2 Tbsp	

Day 5

Food	Serving	Notes
Breakfast		
Organic, Free-Range Chicken Thigh	3 oz	
Sauteed Spinach	1 serving	
Granny Smith Apple	1 apple	
Unrefined Virgin Coconut Oil	1 tsp	
Daily Energy Greens Drink	1 serving	
Morning Snack		
Raw Walnuts	1 oz	
Fresh Mixed Berries	1/2 cup	
Lunch		
Buffalo Meatballs	1 serving	Suggested: Sauté 2 pieces of garlic then add the cut-up tomato. This will serve as the "sauce" for the meatballs. Serve over Spaghetti Squash. (The meatball recipe makes 4 servings. Eat 1 serving for lunch. Share the other servings with family or store in the freezer for another meal.)
Basic Spaghetti Squash	1 serving	
Fresh Tomatoes	1 cup	
Unrefined Virgin Coconut Oil	1 tsp	
Afternoon Snack		
Raw Nut Butter	2 Tbsp	
Fresh Banana	1 banana	
Dinner		
Fresh, Wild-Caught Halibut	5 oz	
Organic Avocado	2 oz	
Organic Broccoli	1 cup	
Super Simple Side Salad	1 salad	
Isabel's Famous Salad Dressing	1-2 Tbsp	

Day 6

Food	Serving	Notes
Breakfast		
Nitrate-Free Organic Bacon	3 oz	
Cage-Free, Organic Eggs	1 egg	
Fresh Tomatoes	1 cup	
Daily Energy Greens Drink	1 serving	
Morning Snack		
Raw Pumpkin Seeds	1 oz	
Granny Smith Apple	1 apple	
Lunch		
Fresh, Wild-Caught Halibut	5 oz	
Organic Broccoli	1 cup	
Organic Avocado	2 oz	
Isabel's Famous Salad Dressing	1-2 Tbsp	
Super Simple Side Salad	1 salad	
Afternoon Snack		
PB&J Spinach Smoothie	1 serving	
Dinner		
Chicken Breast	5 oz	Suggested: Cut up the chicken and veggies and cook in coconut oil to make a stir fry. Add soy sauce to taste. Serve with the salad on the side.
Unrefined Virgin Coconut Oil	2 tsp	
Wheat-Free Soy Sauce	1 tsp	
Organic Zucchini	1/2 cup	
Bell Pepper (any color)	1/2 cup	
Cucumber and Tomato Salad	1 serving	

Day 7 - Free Day

What's a Free Day?

A free day is a strategy we have implemented into the Beyond Diet program to ensure your body continues to lose fat and keep it off for the long term. The free day has been included in these first few weeks of the Beyond Diet program to help you keep your mental focus throughout the entire length of the program as you work towards your goals.

The free day has also been perfectly designed to make the Beyond Diet program a strategy that can be used for a lifetime. The biggest issue people have when "dieting" is that they are unable to sustain the plan for the long term. Not with Beyond Diet. We have planned out every one of your meals so that you are satisfied, full, and happy every step of the way.

Is the free day a cheat day?

We get this question a lot since many diet programs use the words "cheat day." I like the term "free day" much better in that you are not "cheating" at all. There is no cheating on this plan. There are just good choices versus bad choices, and you are free to make any choice you want at any given time.

The meal plans in Beyond Diet make your choices super simple. We give you the exact meals to eat, tell you when to eat them, and give you the shopping lists to go along with it. This strategy has been successful for hundreds of thousands of people over the past 8 years.

But, there are just some days when people do want to make a choice (mostly good choices). Going to a party and you'd rather make the choice? Insert the free day. Going out to dinner and you'd rather make the choice? Yup, you guessed it, free day.

Going to a special event and you want to make a choice? Again, the free day. The free day allows you to make some choices throughout the duration of the program.

How do you implement a free day?

For one out of your three main meals (Breakfast, Lunch, and Dinner), eat absolutely any food you want (yes, I said any food you want). For the other two meals, choose your favorite BD-approved meal from the prior week. For example, if breakfast on Day 3 was your absolute favorite, that will be your breakfast on the free day. If the lunch on Day 5 was your favorite that will be your free day lunch. This allows for dinner to be any meal you want. This would be a good day to go out to dinner and choose your favorite restaurant meal.

You can still have 2 snacks each day. Again, you will choose from your favorite snacks throughout the week. If your meal of choice happens to be a bit larger than you normally would have and you wish to skip your snack, you can do so on the free day (as in example 1).

The free day is designed to make certain situations a bit easier and also to allow you to have some of your favorite meals. Foods I do NOT recommend you have on your free day are fast foods of any kind, processed foods that contain hydrogenated oil and high fructose corn syrup, and deep fried foods in unhealthy vegetable oils. These foods are really just not good during any phase of your healthy eating plan.

Free Day Example #1 – Breakfast Diner Trip

Breakfast – Trip to the diner with the family (I'm from NJ, we like diners) - order of pancakes with whipped cream, fresh fruit, and syrup; coffee with milk or cream

Snack – Possibly decide not to have a snack since still pretty full from breakfast

Lunch – Turkey Chili

Snack – 2 Tbsp almond butter with carrots

Dinner – Day 6 Dinner

Free Day Example #2 – Luncheon with the Family

Breakfast – Day 1 Breakfast

Snack – 1/2 oz pumpkin seeds with small apple

Lunch – Mexican fiesta lunch - 2 hard shell tacos with beef, veggies, and refried beans; a handful of chips with guacamole

Snack – 1/2 oz almonds with 1/2 cup berries

Dinner – Day 2 Dinner

Free Day Example #3 – Dinner Party

Breakfast – Day 1 Breakfast

Snack – 1 oz almonds with 1/2 banana

Lunch – Turkey Chili

Snack – 1 oz almonds with 1/2 banana

Dinner – Appetizers and whatever is served at the party - In situations like these, I try not to be too picky about what I'm eating and just focus on having fun at the party.

Day 8

Food	Serving	Notes
Breakfast		
Cage-Free Organic Eggs	2 eggs	Suggested: Cook the spinach using coconut oil and then add in the eggs (lightly beaten) to make a spinach omelet. Eat over the sliced tomatoes.
Unrefined Virgin Coconut Oil	1 tsp	
Fresh Tomatoes	1 cup	
Fresh Spinach	1 cup	
Daily Energy Greens Drink	1 serving	
Morning Snack		
Raw Almonds	1 oz	
Fresh Banana	1/2 banana	
Lunch		
Fresh, Wild Caught Salmon	4 oz	Suggested: Broil the salmon seasoned with salt and pepper. You can do this the night before to have it ready for today's lunch. Eat it cold over the salad. Eat the broccoli raw or lightly steamed.
Organic Broccoli	1 cup	
Super Simple Side Salad	1 salad	
Isabel's Famous Salad Dressing	1-2 Tbsp	
Afternoon Snack		
Chicken Breast	4 oz	Eat the cauliflower raw or lightly steamed.
Granny Smith Apple	1 apple	
Organic Cauliflower	1 cup	
Dinner		
Turkey Chili	1 serving	This Turkey Chili recipe makes 4 servings. Eat 1 serving for dinner and 1 serving for lunch tomorrow.

Day 9

Food	Serving	Notes
Breakfast		
Sausage (chicken, turkey, or pork)	3 oz	Suggested: Cut up the onions and pepper and cook in coconut oil. Then add in sausage.
Unrefined Virgin Coconut OIl	1 tsp	
Bell Pepper (any color)	1/2 cup	
Onion (any type)	1/2 cup	
Daily Energy Greens Drink	1 serving	
Morning Snack		
Granny Smith Apple	1 apple	
Raw Almonds	1 oz	
Lunch		
Turkey Chili	1 serving	Lunch will be leftovers from last night's dinner.
Afternoon Snack		
Raw Nut Butter	2 Tbsp	
Organic Carrots	1 cup	
Dinner		
Organic, Free-Range Chicken Thigh	4 oz	
Cucumber and Tomato Salad	1 serving	
Isabel's Famous Salad Dressing	1-2 Tbsp	
Garlic Green Beans	1 serving	

Day 10

Food	Serving	Notes
Breakfast		
Nitrate-Free, Organic Bacon	3 oz	
Fresh Tomatoes	1 cup	
Cage-Free Organic Egg	1 egg	
Daily Energy Greens Drink	1 serving	
Morning Snack		
Raw Macadamia Nuts	1/2 oz	
Fresh Mixed Berries	1/2 cup	
Lunch		
Fresh, Wild Caught Salmon	4 oz	Suggested: Cut up the salmon and avocado and add them to the salad.
Organic Avocado	2 oz	
Granny Smith Apple	1 apple	
Super Simple Side Salad	1 salad	
Isabel's Famous Salad Dressing	1-2 Tbsp	
Afternoon Snack		
Fresh Banana	1 banana	
Raw Nut Butter	2 Tbsp	
Dinner		
Turkey Burgers	1 serving	Suggested: Cut up the peppers and onions and saute them in coconut oil. The Turkey Burgers recipe makes 2 burgers - eat 1 for dinner and save the other for tomorrow's lunch.
Sauteed Spinach	1 serving	
Unrefined Virgin Coconut Oil	1 tsp	
Bell Pepper (any color)	1/2 cup	
Onion (any type)	1/2 cup	

Day 11

Food	Serving	Notes
Breakfast		
Cage-Free Organic Egg	2 eggs	Suggested: Hard-boil or soft-boil the eggs. Then cut up the eggs and avocado and serve them over steamed cauliflower.
Organic Cauliflower	1 cup	
Organic Avocado	2 oz	
Daily Energy Greens Drink	1 serving	
Morning Snack		
Raw Nut Butter	2 Tbsp	
Organic Carrots	1 cup	
Lunch		
Turkey Burgers	1 serving	
Celery and Carrots	1 cup	
Granny Smith Apple	1 apple	
Afternoon Snack		
Sliced Turkey	4 oz	
Organic Cucumber	1 cup	
Fresh Tomatoes	1 cup	
Dinner		
Organic, Free-Range Chicken Thigh	4 oz	
Organic Broccoli	1 cup	
Super Simple Side Salad	1 salad	
Isabel's Famous Salad Dressing	1-2 Tbsp	

Day 12

Food	Serving	Notes
Breakfast		
Organic, Free-Range Chicken Thigh	3 oz	
Sauteed Spinach	1 serving	
Unrefined Virgin Coconut Oil	2 tsp	
Granny Smith Apple	1 apple	
Daily Energy Greens Drink	1 serving	
Morning Snack		
Raw Walnuts	1 oz	
Fresh Mixed Berries	1/2 cup	
Lunch		
Buffalo Meatballs	1 serving	Suggested: Saute 2 pieces of garlic and then add the cut-up tomato. This will serve as the "sauce" for the meatballs. Serve over spaghetti squash.
Basic Spaghetti Squash	1 serving	
Fresh Tomatoes	1 cup	
Afternoon Snack		
Fresh Banana	1 banana	
Raw Nut Butter	2 Tbsp	
Dinner		
Fresh, Wild-Caught Halibut	5 oz	
Organic Broccoli	1 cup	
Organic Avocado	2 oz	
Super Simple Side Salad	1 salad	
Isabel's Famous Salad Dressing	1-2 Tbsp	

Day 13

Food	Serving	Notes
Breakfast		
Nitrate-Free Organic Bacon	3 oz	
Fresh Tomatoes	1 cup	
Cage-Free Organic Egg	1 egg	
Daily Energy Greens Drink	1 serving	
Morning Snack		
Raw Pumpkin Seeds	1 oz	
Granny Smith Apple	1 apple	
Lunch		
Fresh, Wild-Caught Halibut	5 oz	
Organic Broccoli	1 cup	
Organic Avocado	2 oz	
Super Simple Side Salad	1 salad	
Isabel's Famous Salad Dressing	1-2 Tbsp	
Afternoon Snack		
Sliced Turkey	4 oz	
Granny Smith Apple	1 apple	
Organic Romaine Lettuce	1 cup	
Dinner		
Chicken Breast	5 oz	Suggested: Cut up the chicken and veggies and cook in coconut oil to make stir fry. Add soy sauce to taste. Serve with salad on the side.
Unrefined Virgin Coconut Oil	1 tsp	
Wheat-Free Soy Sauce	1 tsp	
Bell Pepper (any color)	1/2 cup	
Organic Zucchini	1/2 cup	
Cucumber and Tomato Salad	1 serving	

Day 14 - Free Day

See Day 7 for more information on how to handle a free day.

Congratulations! You have completed the first 14 Days of Supercharged Meal Plans.

The next step on your health and weight loss journey is outlined for you in the Beyond Diet Program Guide (on page 10).

Recipes

Isabel's Famous Salad Dressing

16 Servings, 0 Proteins/1 Fat/0 Carbs

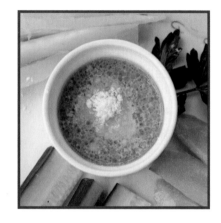

- 1 tsp dijon mustard
- 1/2 tsp garlic powder
- 1/2 tsp unrefined sea salt
- 1/4 cup apple cider vinegar
- 3/4 cup extra virgin olive oil
- 2 Tbsp Parmesan cheese

Combine all ingredients in a salad shaker, and shake well! The apple cider vinegar is the "magic ingredient," but the olive oil is the main ingredient and will make up most of the dressing. Enjoy!

Super Simple Side Salad

1 Serving, 0 Proteins/0 Fats/2 Carbs

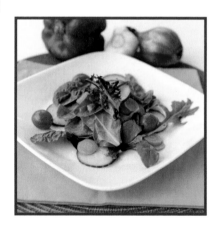

- 1 cup mixed greens
- 1 small carrot
- 1/2 small zucchini
- 1/2 handful cherry tomatoes

Cut carrot and zucchini (or use a cucumber) into small rounds, or peel with a julienne peeler. Toss all ingredients together and add Isabel's Famous Salad Dressing.

Turkey Chili

4 servings, 4 Proteins/0 Fats/1 Carb

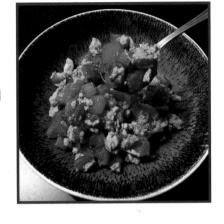

2 tsp (10mL) butter, divided
2 tsp (10mL) chili powder
1 lb (450g) lean ground turkey
1 cup (150g) coarsely chopped red
     bell pepper
1 medium onion, coarsely
     chopped (~¾ cup (120g)
1 bay leaf
1 clove garlic, minced
1 tsp (5mL) paprika
1 tsp (5mL) ground cumin
Dash ground cayenne pepper
14 ½ oz (400g) plum tomatoes, chopped (canned with juice is fine)
½ cup (120mL) chicken stock (or low-fat low-sodium chicken broth)
2/3 cup (100g) coarsely chopped celery (~2/3 stalk)
salt and freshly ground black pepper to taste

Heat 1 tsp (5mL) butter in a 3-quart saucepan over high heat. Add the turkey, and season to taste with the salt and black pepper. Break up the turkey and cook for 2–3 minutes, or until browned. Remove to a bowl and cover to keep warm.

Reduce the heat to low, heat the other 1 tsp butter, and cook the red pepper, onion, celery, and garlic for 3–5 minutes, or until vegetables begin to soften. Add the chili powder, paprika, cumin, and cayenne and cook, stirring, for 1 minute. Increase the heat to medium, and add the tomatoes, stock, and bay leaf. Bring to a boil over high heat. Reduce the heat to medium-low, and simmer uncovered for 15 minutes.

Add the browned turkey, and simmer 5 minutes more. Remove and discard the bay leaf before serving.

Cucumber and Tomato Salad

1 Serving, 0 Proteins/0 Fats/1 Carb

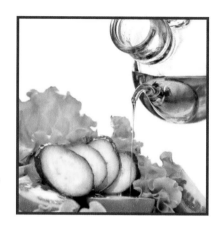

- 1 medium tomato
- 1/2 cucumber
- 1/2 Tbsp fresh basil
- 1/2 Tbsp fresh parsley

Chop all of the vegetables and combine all ingredients in a large bowl, and toss well. Add whatever salad dressing you choose.

Garlic Green Beans

1 Serving, 0 Proteins/0 Fats/2 Carbs

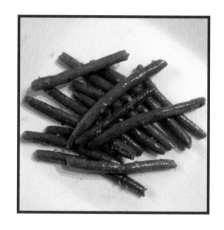

- 1 cup green beans
- 1 tsp coconut oil
- 1-2 garlic cloves
- Sea salt and pepper, to taste

Heat coconut oil in a skillet over medium-high heat. Add minced garlic (1-2 cloves, depending on your taste) and green beans, and sauté until crisp tender. Season green beans with salt and pepper, and reduce heat to medium. Cover skillet and let steam for 2-3 minutes, stirring occasionally. If you desire, you may steam for as long as 10 minutes – this will give the green beans a very soft, delicate flavor.

Sautéed Spinach

1 Serving, 0 Proteins/0 Fats/1 Carb

2 cups fresh spinach
1 tsp coconut oil
2 garlic cloves
Sea salt and pepper, to taste

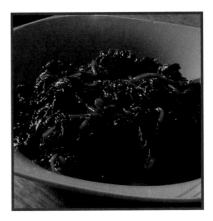

Heat coconut oil and garlic in a skillet on low to medium heat. Add spinach and heat until wilted. Remove from heat. Add salt, pepper, and any other seasonings you choose.

Turkey Burgers

2 Servings, 4 Proteins/0 Fats/0 Carbs

1/2 lb ground turkey
1/2 tsp sea salt
1/2 tsp black pepper
1/2 tsp paprika
1/4 tsp garlic powder
1/4 tsp cayenne pepper

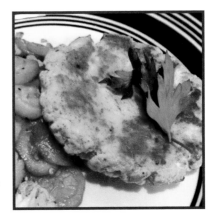

Mix together salt, pepper, paprika, garlic powder, and cayenne pepper (if you don't like these seasonings, you can use different ones). In a bowl, use your hands to mix ground turkey with seasonings. Form mixture into 2 patties. Cook on a grill or in a pan on the stove top.

Basic Spaghetti Squash

6 Servings, 0 Proteins/1 Fat/1 Carb

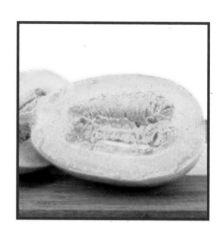

  1 medium spaghetti squash
  2 Tbsp unsalted butter
  Sea salt and pepper, to taste

Preheat oven to 350°F. Cut spaghetti squash in half lengthwise; remove and discard seeds. Place squash, cut sides down, in a baking pan with about 1/2 inch of water. Bake for about 1 hour, or until tender when pricked with a fork.

Let squash cool slightly, then remove the strands of flesh, bit by bit, with a fork. Mix in butter, salt, and pepper.

Variation: Serve topped with grated Parmesan cheese, pesto, or tomato sauce.

Depending on the size of the spaghetti squash, you may get anywhere from 4-8 servings.

Buffalo Meatballs

4 Servings, 4 Proteins/0 Fats/0 Carbs

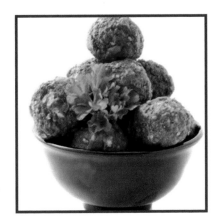

  1 lb ground buffalo
  1 1/2 tsp garlic powder
  1 1/2 tsp oregano
  1 1/2 tsp parsley
  1 tsp thyme
  Sea salt and pepper, to taste

Combine all ingredients in a bowl, and use your hands to mix. Form mixture into meatballs, and cook for 40-45 minutes in a 375°F oven.

PB&J Spinach Smoothie

1 Serving, 2 Proteins/0 Fats/2 Carbs

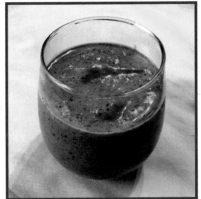

  1/2 med banana, frozen
  1/2 cup mixed berries, frozen
  2 Tbsp almond butter
  1 cup spinach
  1/4 cup water

Combine all ingredients in a blender, and blend until smooth.

No frozen bananas? Use a fresh one, and add ice cubes to the blender.

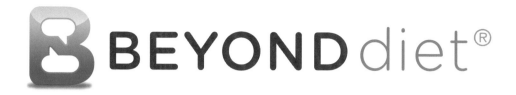

DAYS 15-28 OF

SUPERCHARGED MEAL PLANS

Isabel De Los Rios

Introduction

Congratulations! You've completed the first phase of 14 Days of Supercharged Meal Plans. Chances are you are already experiencing great results after those first two weeks. Isn't it such a great feeling? Are you ready to embark on the next two weeks of the Beyond Diet program?

This next set of meal plans will help you continue to see more of the progress and results you saw during the first two weeks. These meal plans will also introduce you to some basic and easy cooking methods. Even the most beginner cook in the kitchen will absolutely love putting together these meals. That's one of the great side benefits of the Beyond Diet program... people start to use their kitchens more, and they love the meals they create! (And, just like the first two weeks, the meals will continue to be flavorful and filling so you are not battling any cravings during the day.)

If there is a meal that you don't particularly like, or a meal that contains a food you cannot eat for any reason, you can always repeat another meal from that same category. For example, if you do not like eggs or are allergic to them, you can make one of the smoothie options for breakfast instead. You can also use one of the meals from the first set of 14 Day Meal Plans. Some of those meals are my go-to favorites for breakfast and lunch as well as the ones you will see here.

Grocery Shopping Guide

Week 1 – Days 1 through 6

(*Some products purchased during week 1 will be left over to use for week 2)

Produce	Amount	Notes
Apples (Green)	4	3 red + 1 Granny Smith
Asparagus	4 cups	
Avocados	2	
Bananas	4	
Bell Peppers	4-5	Any color - Make sure 2 are red
Berries	2 cups	Any berries - strawberries, blueberries, raspberries, blackberries.
Carrots	11	
Cauliflower	1 head	
Celery	1 cup	
Cherry Tomatoes	2 1/2 cups	
Garlic	1 head	
Greens (mixed)	3 cups	Romaine, Arugula, Red Leaf, or Bibb Lettuce
Jalapeño Pepper	1	
Lemons	2	
Limes	2	
Mushrooms (white)	1/4 cup	
Onions	4	Make sure 2 are yellow, 1 is white
Peaches	2	
Spaghetti Squash	1	

Produce (cont.)	Amount	Notes
Spinach	3 1/2 cups	
Tomatoes (diced)	1/4 cup	
Zucchini	5	
Meat & Seafood	**Amount**	**Notes**
Chicken Breast	1 1/2 pounds	Free-Range
Ground Beef	1 pound	Grass-Fed
Ground Turkey	1 1/2 pounds	Free-Range
Salmon	10 ounces	2 fillets
Sliced Turkey	6 ounces	Nitrate-Free
Eggs & Dairy	**Amount**	**Notes**
Butter		Grass-fed, Organic
Eggs	14	Cage-Free, Organic
Parmesan Cheese		
Nuts & Seeds	**Amount**	**Notes**
Almond Flour	2 cups	
Almond Milk	1 1/2 cups	
Coconut Flour	1/4 cup	
Coconut Milk	1/4 cup	
Nut Butter	1 jar	Almond Butter, Cashew Butter, or Walnut Butter
Raw Walnuts	7 ounces	
Miscellaneous	**Amount**	**Notes**
Apple Cider Vinegar	1/4 cup	
Baking Soda		Aluminum-free
Chicken Broth	2 cups	
Chickpeas	1 cup	

Miscellaneous (cont.)	Amount	Notes
Coconut Oil	1 jar	
Daily Energy	1	http://go.beyonddiet.com/DailyEnergy
Dijon Mustard		
Extra Virgin Olive Oil		
Maple Syrup		Pure, Grade B
Soy Sauce		Wheat-Free
Tahini	1/2 cup	
Tomato Sauce	1/4 cup	
Vanilla Extract		
Seasonings	Amount	Notes
Basil (dried)		
Black Pepper		
Cayenne Pepper		
Cinnamon		
Cumin		
Garlic Powder		
Nutmeg		
Oregano (dried)		
Paprika		
Parsley (dried)		
Red Pepper Flakes		
Sea Salt		http://go.beyonddiet.com/AztecSeaSalt

Week 2 – Days 8 through 13

Produce	Amount	Notes
Apples	4	3 red + 1 Granny Smith
Asparagus	2 cups	
Avocados	2	
Bananas	4	
Bell Peppers	4-5	Any color - make sure 2 are red
Berries	2 cups	Any berries - strawberries, blueberries, raspberries, blackberries.
Carrots	12	
Cauliflower	1	Medium
Celery	1 cup	
Cherry Tomatoes	2 1/2 cups	
Garlic	1 head	
Greens (mixed)	3 cups	Romaine, Arugula, Red Leaf, or Bibb Lettuce
Jalapeño Pepper	1	
Lemons	2	
Limes	2	
Mushrooms (white)	1/4 cup	
Onions	4	Make sure 2 are yellow, 1 is white
Peaches	2	
Spaghetti Squash	1	
Spinach	1 1/2 cups	
Tomatoes (diced)	1/4 cup	
Zucchini	5	

Meat & Seafood	Amount	Notes
Chicken Breast	1 pound	Free-Range
Ground Beef	1 pound	Grass-Fed
Ground Turkey	1/2 pound	Free-Range
Salmon	10 ounces	2 fillets
Sliced Turkey	6 ounces	
Eggs & Dairy	**Amount**	**Notes**
Eggs	13	Cage-Free, Organic
Nuts & Seeds	**Amount**	**Notes**
Almond Flour	1 1/2 cups	
Almond Milk	1 1/2 cups	
Coconut Flour	1/4 cup	
Coconut Milk	1/4 cup	
Raw Walnuts	7 ounces	
Miscellaneous	**Amount**	**Notes**
Chicken Broth	1 1/2 cups	
Chickpeas	1 cup	
Tahini	1/4 cup	
Tomato Sauce	1/4 cup	

Day 1

Food	Serving	Notes
Breakfast		
Spinach Mushroom Omelet	1 serving	
Red Apple	1 apple	
Daily Energy Greens Drink	1 serving	
Morning Snack		
Fresh Peach	1 peach	
Raw Walnuts	1 ounce	
Lunch		
Sauteed Chicken with Asparagus and Peppers	1 serving	
Simple Side Salad	1 salad	
Isabel's Famous Salad Dressing	1-2 Tbsp	
Afternoon Snack		
Sliced Turkey	2 ounces	
Organic Carrots	1 cup	
Dinner		
Turkey and Spinach Meatballs	1 serving	
Zucchini Pasta	1 serving	

Day 2

Food	Serving	Notes
Breakfast		
Apple, Almond, and Avocado Smoothie	1 serving	
Egg Spinach Scramble	1 serving	
Daily Energy Greens Drink	1 serving	
Morning Snack		
Sliced Turkey	2 oz	
Organic Carrots	1 cup	
Lunch		
Turkey and Spinach Meatballs	1 serving	
Zucchini Pasta	1 serving	
Afternoon Snack		
Hard-Boiled Eggs	1 egg	
Bell Pepper (any color)	1 cup	
Dinner		
Well-Seasoned Meatloaf	1 serving	
Garlicky Mashed Cauliflower	1 serving	

Day 3

Food	Serving	Notes
Breakfast		
Gluten Free Coconut Flour Pancakes	1 serving	
Daily Energy Greens Drink	1 serving	
Morning Snack		
Red Apple	1 apple	
Raw Nut Butter	2 Tbsp	
Lunch		
Well-Seasoned Meatloaf	1 serving	
Garlicky Mashed Cauliflower	1 serving	
Afternoon Snack		
Sliced Turkey	2 oz	
Organic Carrots·	1 cup	
Dinner		
Savory Salmon	1 serving	
Basic Spaghetti Squash	1 serving	

Day 4

Food	Serving	Notes
Breakfast		
Zucchini Omelet	1 serving	
Granny Smith Apple	1 apple	
Daily Energy Greens Drink	1 serving	
Morning Snack		
Traditional Hummus	1 serving	
Celery and Carrots	1 cup	
Lunch		
Savory Salmon	1 serving	
Basic Spaghetti Squash	1 serving	
Afternoon Snack		
Raw Walnuts	1 oz	
Fresh Mixed Berries	1 cup	
Dinner		
Mexican Lime Chicken Soup	1 serving	

Day 5

Food	Serving	Notes
Breakfast		
Banana Almond Butter Smoothie	1 serving	
Daily Energy Greens Drink	1 serving	
Morning Snack		
Raw Walnuts	1 oz	
Fresh Mixed Berries	1 cup	
Lunch		
Mexican Lime Chicken Soup	1 serving	
Afternoon Snack		
Hard-Boiled Eggs	1 egg	
Bell Pepper (any color)	1 cup	
Dinner		
Turkey Burgers	1 burger	
The Best Carrot Fries	1 serving	
Super Simple Side Salad	1 salad	
Isabel's Famous Salad Dressing	1-2 Tbsp	

Day 6

Food	Serving	Notes
Breakfast		
Banana Walnut Muffins	1 serving	
Daily Energy Greens Drink	1 serving	
Morning Snack		
Fresh Peach	1 peach	
Raw Nut Butter	2 Tbsp	
Lunch		
Turkey Burgers	1 burger	
The Best Carrot Fries	1 serving	
Afternoon Snack		
Traditional Hummus	1 serving	
Celery and Carrots	1 cup	
Dinner		
Sautéed Chicken with Asparagus and Peppers	1 serving	
Simple Side Salad	1 salad	
Isabel's Famous Salad Dressing	1-2 Tbsp	

Day 7 - Free Day

What's a Free Day?

A free day is a strategy we have implemented into the Beyond Diet program to ensure your body continues to lose fat and keep it off for the long term. The free day has been included in these first few weeks of the Beyond Diet program to help you keep your mental focus throughout the entire length of the program as you work towards your goal.

The free day has also been perfectly designed to make the Beyond Diet program a strategy that can be used for a lifetime. The biggest issue people have when "dieting" is that they are unable to sustain the plan for the long term. Not with Beyond Diet. We have planned out every one of your meals so that you are satisfied, full, and happy every step of the way.

Is the free day a cheat day?

We get this question a lot since many diet programs use the words "cheat day." I like the term "free day" much better in that you are not "cheating" at all. There is no cheating on this plan. There are just good choices versus bad choices, and you are free to make any choice you want at any given time.

The meal plans in Beyond Diet make your choices super simple. We give you the exact meals to eat, tell you when to eat them, and give you the shopping lists to go along with it. This strategy has been successful for hundreds of thousands of people over the past 8 years.

But, there are just some days when people do want to make a choice (mostly good choices). Going to a party and you'd rather make the choice? Insert the free day. Going out to dinner and you'd rather make the choice? Yup, you guessed it, free day.

Going to a special event and you want to make a choice? Again, the free day. The free day allows you to make some choices throughout the duration of the program.

How do you implement a free day?

For one out of your three main meals (Breakfast, Lunch and Dinner), eat absolutely any food you want (yes, I said any food you want). For the other two meals, choose your favorite BD-approved meal from the prior week. For example, if breakfast on Day 3 was your absolute favorite, that will be your breakfast on the free day. If the lunch on Day 5 was your favorite that will be your free day lunch. This allows for dinner to be any meal you want. This would be a good day to go out to dinner and choose your favorite restaurant meals.

You can still have 2 snacks each day. Again, you will choose from your favorite snacks throughout the week. If your meal of choice happens to be a bit larger than you normally would have and you wish to skip your snack, you can do so on the free day (as in example 1).

The free day is designed to make certain situations a bit easier and also to allow you to have some of your favorite meals. Foods I do NOT recommend you have on your free day are fast foods of any kind, processed foods that contain hydrogenated oil and high fructose corn syrup, and deep fried foods in unhealthy vegetable oils. These foods are really just not good during any phase of your healthy eating plan.

Day 8

Food	Serving	Notes
Breakfast		
Spinach Mushroom Omelet	1 serving	
Red Apple	1 apple	
Daily Energy Greens Drink	1 serving	
Morning Snack		
Fresh Peach	1 peach	
Raw Walnuts	1 oz	
Lunch		
Sauteed Chicken with Asparagus and Peppers	1 serving	
Simple Side Salad	1 serving	
Isabel's Famous Salad Dressing	1-2 Tbsp	
Afternoon Snack		
Sliced Turkey	2 oz	
Organic Carrots	1 cup	
Dinner		
Turkey and Spinach Meatballs	1 serving	
Zucchini Pasta	1 serving	

Day 9

Food	Serving	Notes
Breakfast		
Apple, Almond, and Avocado Smoothie	1 serving	
Egg Spinach Scramble	1 serving	
Daily Energy Greens Drink	1 serving	
Morning Snack		
Sliced Turkey	2 oz	
Organic Carrots	1 cup	
Lunch		
Turkey and Spinach Meatballs	1 serving	
Zucchini Pasta	1 serving	
Afternoon Snack		
Hard-Boiled Eggs	1 egg	
Bell Pepper (any color)	1 cup	
Dinner		
Well-Seasoned Meatloaf	1 serving	
Garlicky Mashed Cauliflower	1 serving	

Day 10

Food	Serving	Notes
Breakfast		
Gluten Free Coconut Flour Pancakes	1 serving	
Daily Energy Greens Drink	1 serving	
Morning Snack		
Red Apple	1 apple	
Raw Nut Butter	2 Tbsp	
Lunch		
Well-Seasoned Meatloaf	1 serving	
Garlicky Mashed Cauliflower	1 serving	
Afternoon Snack		
Sliced Turkey	2 oz	
Organic Carrots	1 cup	
Dinner		
Savory Salmon	1 serving	
Basic Spaghetti Squash	1 serving	

Day 11

Food	Serving	Notes
Breakfast		
Zucchini Omelet	1 serving	
Granny Smith Apple	1 apple	
Daily Energy Greens Drink	1 serving	
Morning Snack		
Traditional Hummus	1 serving	
Celery and Carrots	1 cup	
Lunch		
Savory Salmon	1 serving	
Basic Spaghetti Squash	1 serving	
Afternoon Snack		
Raw Walnuts	1 oz	
Fresh Mixed Berries	1 cup	
Dinner		
Mexican Lime Chicken Soup	1 serving	

Day 12

Food	Serving	Notes
Breakfast		
Banana Almond Butter Smoothie	1 serving	
Daily Energy Greens Drink	1 serving	
Morning Snack		
Raw Walnuts	1 oz	
Fresh Mixed Berries	1 cup	
Lunch		
Mexican Lime Chicken Soup	1 serving	
Afternoon Snack		
Hard-Boiled Eggs	1 egg	
Bell Pepper (any color)	1 cup	
Dinner		
Turkey Burgers	1 burger	
The Best Carrot Fries	1 serving	
Simple Side Salad	1 salad	
Isabel's Famous Salad Dressing	1-2 Tbsp	

Day 13

Food	Serving	Notes
Breakfast		
Banana Walnut Muffins	1 serving	
Daily Energy Greens Drink	1 serving	
Morning Snack		
Fresh Peach	1 peach	
Raw Nut Butter	2 Tbsp	
Lunch		
Turkey Burgers	1 burger	
The Best Carrot Fries	1 serving	
Afternoon Snack		
Traditional Hummus	1 serving	
Celery and Carrots	1 cup	
Dinner		
Sautéed Chicken with Asparagus and Peppers	1 serving	
Simple Side Salad	1 salad	
Isabel's Famous Salad Dressing	1-2 Tbsp	

Day 14 - Free Day

See Day 7 for more information on how to handle a free day.

Congratulations! You have completed the first 4 weeks of the Beyond Diet program!

Ready for the next step? Check out the Beyond Diet Program Guide (on page 10) to see what's next on your health and weight loss journey.

Recipes

Spinach Mushroom Omelet

1 Serving, 2 Proteins/0 Fats/1 Carb

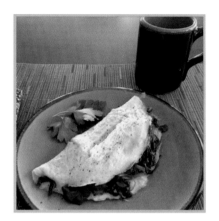

    2 eggs
    1/2 cup fresh spinach
    1/4 cup mushrooms
    2 Tbsp onion, any type
    1 Tbsp bell pepper, any color
    1/4 cup tomatoes, diced
    1 tsp coconut oil
    Sea salt and pepper, to taste
    Red pepper flakes, to taste
    Garlic Powder, to taste

Whisk eggs in a small bowl. Mix in seasonings.

Heat coconut oil in a skillet over medium heat. Add sliced mushrooms, diced onion, and chopped bell pepper to skillet. Cook until veggies are tender, about 5 minutes.

Add spinach to skillet, and cook until wilted. Stir in diced tomatoes and egg mixture. As the egg mixture sets, lift the edges to allow the uncooked portion to flow underneath.

Cook until the egg mixture sets, about 10-15 minutes.

Super Simple Side Salad

1 Serving, 0 Proteins/0 Fats/2 Carbs

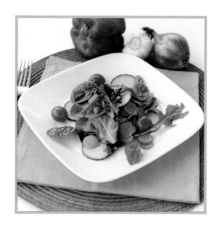

1 cup mixed greens
1 small carrot
1/2 small zucchini
1/2 handful cherry tomatoes

Cut carrot and zucchini (or use a cucumber) into small rounds, or peel with a julienne peeler. Toss all ingredients together and add Isabel's Famous Salad Dressing.

Isabel's Famous Salad Dressing

16 servings, 0 Proteins/1 Fat/0 Carbs

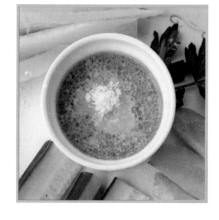

1 tsp dijon mustard
1/2 tsp garlic powder
1/2 tsp unrefined sea salt
1/4 cup apple cider vinegar
3/4 cup extra virgin olive oil
2 Tbsp Parmesan cheese

Combine all ingredients in a salad shaker, and shake well! The apple cider vinegar is the "magic ingredient," but the olive oil is the main ingredient and will make up most of the dressing. Enjoy!

Sautéed Chicken with Asparagus and Peppers

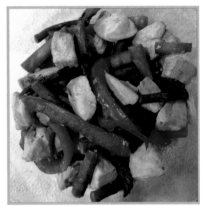

2 Servings, 4 Proteins/0 Fats/2 Carbs

   1 medium onion, any type
   1 clove garlic
   1 Tbsp chicken broth
   1/2 lb chicken breast
   1/2 medium bell pepper, red
   2 cups asparagus, fresh
   2 Tbsp soy sauce
   Sea salt and pepper, to taste

Put chicken broth in a skillet over medium-high heat. Add onions (cut in half and into slices) and peppers (cut into slices) and sauté for about 2 minutes, stirring constantly. Add minced garlic and chicken (cut into bite-sized pieces) and soy sauce. Stir it all up, and cover. Cook for 2-3 minutes, until asparagus is tender.

Zucchini Pasta

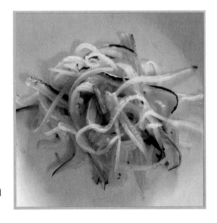

1 Serving, 0 Proteins/0 Fats/2 Carbs

   1 medium zucchini
   1/2 cup cherry tomatoes
   2 tsp coconut oil
   Sea salt and pepper, to taste

Peel zucchini using a julienne peeler, or create "noodles" using a spiralizer. Heat oil in a skillet over medium heat. Add "noodles" and halved cherry tomatoes, and cook until heated through. Season with salt and pepper.

Apple, Almond, and Avocado Smoothie

1 Serving, 1 Protein/2 Fats/2 Carbs

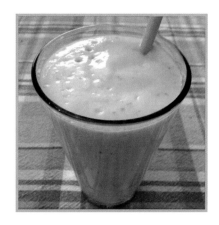

   1 medium red apple
   1/2 medium avocado
   1 cup almond milk
   1/2 medium banana
   1/2 cup ice

Combine all ingredients in a blender, and blend until smooth.

Egg Spinach Scramble

1 Serving, 1 Protein/0 Fats/1 Carb

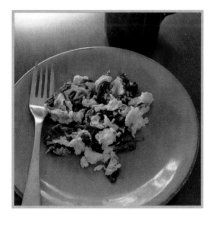

   1 egg
   1 cup spinach
   1 tsp coconut oil

Heat a skillet over medium heat. Add coconut oil and let warm for 30 seconds. Add spinach and let wilt. Add egg and scramble into the spinach.

Well-Seasoned Meatloaf

5 Servings, 4 Proteins/0 Fats/0 Carbs

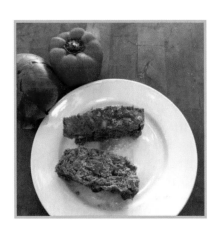

1 lb ground beef
1 medium yellow onion
1 roasted red pepper
1/4 cup tomato sauce
3/4 cup almond flour
1 egg
1 tsp basil
1 tsp parsley
1 tsp oregano
Sea salt and pepper, to taste
1 Tbsp coconut oil

Preheat oven to 400°F. Heat coconut oil in a skillet over medium heat. Add diced onion and diced roasted red pepper to the pan. Cook until onions are soft and translucent.

Combine all other ingredients in a bowl. Add onions and peppers to the bowl when they are done cooking and cooled. Use your hands to mix it all together.

Transfer mixture into a loaf pan. Bake for 35-40 minutes.

After it has cooled a bit, cut your meatloaf into 5 even pieces. Eat 1 serving for dinner and save 1 serving for tomorrow's lunch. If you are not also feeding other family members, you can freeze the remaining 3 servings to be used next week.

Garlicky Mashed Cauliflower

4 Servings, 0 Proteins/1 Fat/1 Carb

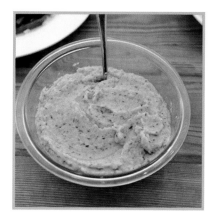

- 1 medium cauliflower
- 1 small yellow onion
- 2 Tbsp butter
- 2 garlic cloves

Separate cauliflower into florets, and steam or boil it. Chop the onion and sauté it with either olive oil, butter, or coconut oil. (My sister used olive oil. I use butter).

Add the cooked cauliflower to the sautéed onions and sauté together for approximately 8 minutes. Take the cauliflower and onion sauté and puree in a food processor or blender. Add a tablespoon or more of butter and blend.

Take 2 cloves of garlic and chop them up into small pieces. Add more olive oil, butter or coconut oil to pan and cook the garlic until brown (but try not to burn it). Pour the garlic into your mashed cauliflower and mix by hand.

Gluten Free Coconut Flour Pancakes

2 Servings, 2 Proteins/0 Fats/1 Carb

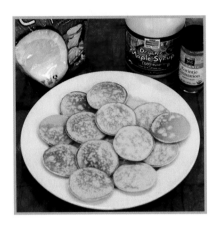

  4 eggs
  1/4 cup coconut flour
  1/4 cup coconut milk
  1 Tbsp maple syrup
  1/4 tsp vanilla extract
  1 pinch nutmeg
  1 pinch cinnamon

In a large bowl, whisk the eggs really well. Sift in the coconut flour, and quickly whisk to mix well. Add coconut milk, and continue to mix well.

Optional: Stir in the maple syrup (or use raw honey) and seasonings.

Use butter to grease griddle at 325°F or pan over medium heat. Pour about 1/4 cup of batter onto the griddle for each pancake, allowing each side to brown before flipping it. (Watch carefully so they don't burn!)

Savory Salmon

1 Serving, 4 Proteins/1 Fat/0 Carbs

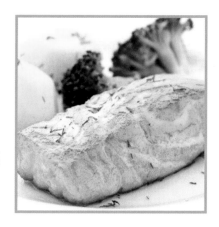

    5 oz salmon
    3/4 tsp garlic powder
    3/4 tsp basil
    1 tsp butter
    Sea salt and pepper, to taste

Combine garlic powder, basil, and salt in a small bowl. Rub onto the fillet.

Melt butter in a skillet over medium heat. Cook salmon in butter until browned and flaky, about 5 minutes per side.

Zucchini Omelet

1 Serving, 2 Proteins/0 Fats/1 Carb

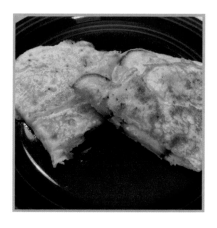

    2 eggs
    1 cup zucchini
    Sea salt and pepper, to taste
    1 tsp coconut oil

Heat a little coconut oil in a small skillet over medium heat. Whisk eggs in a small bowl. Season with salt and pepper. Pour eggs into skillet and let cook.

Arrange zucchini slices on half of the egg. When eggs have set, use a spatula to fold in half.

Continue to cook, letting the insides completely cook through.

Basic Spaghetti Squash

6 Servings, 0 Proteins/1 Fat/1 Carb

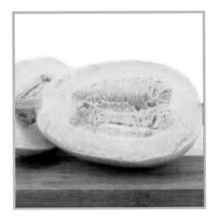

   1 medium spaghetti squash
   2 Tbsp butter
   Sea salt and pepper, to taste

Preheat oven to 350°F. Cut
spaghetti squash in half
lengthwise; remove and discard
seeds.

Place squash, cut sides down, in a
baking pan with about 1/2 inch of water. Bake for about 1 hour,
or until tender when pricked with a fork.

Let squash cool slightly, then remove the strands of flesh, bit by
bit, with a fork.

Mix in butter, salt, and pepper.

Variation: Serve topped with grated Parmesan cheese, pesto, or
tomato sauce.

Depending on the size of the spaghetti squash, you may get
anywhere from 4-8 servings.

Traditional Hummus

10 Servings, 0 Proteins/0 Fats/0 Carb

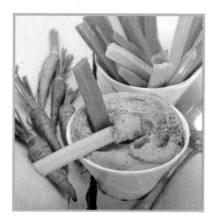

  1 cup chickpeas, dry
  3 1/4 tsp baking soda
  1/2 cup tahini
  3 Tbsp lemon juice
  2 garlic cloves
  1/2 tsp cumin powder
  Sea salt, to taste

Rinse chickpeas in a colander several times until the water runs clear. Place the clean beans in a large bowl (at least 3 times the volume of the beans), add 3 teaspoons of baking soda, and fill bowl with water. Place this bowl in the refrigerator and soak the beans overnight.

The next morning, drain the beans, refill the bowl with water, and soak a couple more hours. Rinse the beans one more time, then place in a large pot.

Cover the beans with water, add 1/4 teaspoon of baking soda (do not add salt), and cook beans until easily mashed between fingers, about 1 to 1 1/2 hours. (Alternatively, you could place the beans in a crockpot and cook on high for about 4 to 6 hours.)

Once cooked, sieve the beans, reserving the cooking water.

Puree the beans in a food processor until very smooth. Let that cool for a while before proceeding.

Once cool, add tahini, lemon juice, chopped garlic, cumin, and salt to the beans in the food processor. At this point you can adjust the ingredients to your taste, adding more of the items listed or something new.

If the hummus is too thick, add little bits of the cooking water until desired consistency is reached. You do want it to be thinner than the desired end result (it will thicken in the fridge).

Serving suggestion: drizzle with a bit of good olive oil and sprinkle with chopped parsley.

Mexican Lime Chicken Soup

2 Servings, 4 Proteins/2 Fats/0 Carbs

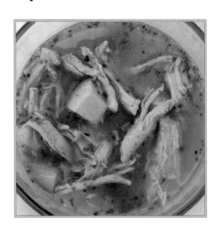

2 limes
1/2 lb chicken breast
1/2 tsp sea salt
1/4 tsp black pepper
2 tsp coconut oil
1/2 white onion
3 garlic cloves
1 jalapeño
1 1/2 cups chicken broth
1 1/2 cups water
1 tsp oregano
1 medium avocado

Season chicken breasts with salt and pepper.

Heat coconut oil in a large saucepan over medium heat. Add chicken and cook until browned, about 5 minute. Remove the chicken from the pan (put on a plate).

Add chopped onion to the pan and sauté until translucent, about 4 minutes. Add minced garlic and minced jalapeño and sauté until fragrant, about 1 minute.

Add chicken broth, water, fresh squeezed lime juice (from 1 lime), and oregano.

Put the chicken back in the pan. Turn up the heat to high; bring the liquid to a boil. Skim off any foam that rises to the surface.

When the liquid boils, reduce heat to medium low, cover partially, and simmer for 30 minutes

Remove the chicken from the pan, letting the soup continue to simmer. Shred the chicken into bite-size pieces, and stir it back into the soup.

To serve: Put diced avocado and a couple lime wedges in a bowl. Ladle the soup into the bowl and enjoy!

Banana Almond Butter Smoothie

1 Serving, 2 Proteins/0 Fats/2 Carbs

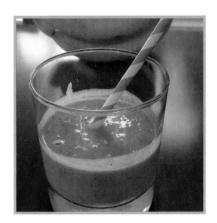

> 1 medium banana, frozen
> 2 Tbsp almond butter
> 1/2 tsp vanilla extract
> 1/2 cup almond milk

Preheat oven to 350°F. Cut Combine banana, almond butter, and vanilla in a blender. Blend until smooth, adding almond milk as needed to reach desired consistency.

If you don't have a frozen banana, use a fresh one and add some ice to the blender.

Turkey Burgers

2 Servings, 4 Proteins/0 Fats/0 Carbs

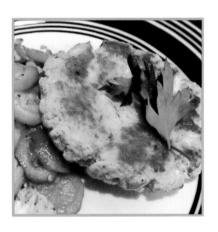

> 1/2 lb ground turkey
> 1/2 tsp sea salt
> 1/2 tsp paprika
> 1/4 tsp garlic powder
> 1/4 tsp cayenne pepper

Mix together salt, pepper, paprika, garlic powder, and cayenne pepper (if you don't like these seasonings, you can use different ones).

In a bowl, use your hands to mix ground turkey with seasonings. Form mixture into 2 patties. Cook on a grill or in a pan on the stove top.

The Best Carrot Fries

4 Servings, 0 Proteins/0 Fats/1 Carb

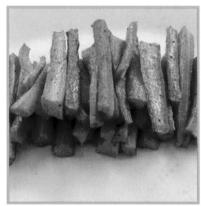

- 1 lb carrots
- 1 Tbsp coconut oil
- 1/2 tsp sea salt
- 1/2 tsp black pepper

Preheat oven to 350ºF. Line a baking sheet with parchment paper.

Wash, peel, and cut carrots into 1/2-inch sticks. Put carrots in a bowl, drizzle with oil, sprinkle with salt and pepper, and toss to coat.

Arrange carrot sticks in a single layer on baking sheet. Bake for 10-15 minutes, turning halfway through.

Banana Walnut Muffins

4 Servings, 2 Proteins/0 Fats/1 Carb

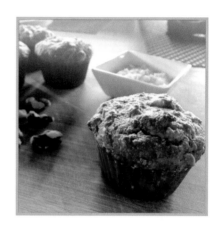

- 2 1/2 medium bananas
- 1 Tbsp coconut oil
- 1 egg
- 1 1/2 cups almond flour
- 1 pinch sea salt
- 1/2 tsp baking soda
- 1/2 cup walnuts

Preheat oven to 350°F. Line 8 muffin cups with liners. Mash the bananas in a bowl (very ripe bananas are best for this recipe). Add coconut oil and eggs, and blend until mixture is smooth. Add almond flour, salt and baking soda, and mix well. Add the walnuts, and stir to combine.

Spoon the batter into muffin cups. Bake for 20-25 minutes, or until the muffins are golden brown and a toothpick inserted in the center of a muffin comes out clean. Let muffins cool in the pan for about half an hour, then serve. Two muffins are one serving.

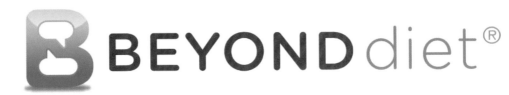

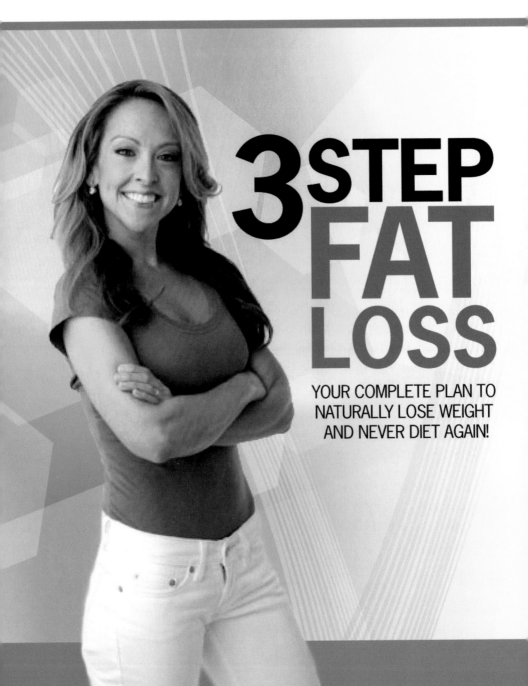

3STEP FAT LOSS

YOUR COMPLETE PLAN TO
NATURALLY LOSE WEIGHT
AND NEVER DIET AGAIN!

1: A Program for Success

Achieving success in any weight loss program takes more than just following nutritional information; it requires getting into the right state of mind. All of our actions are governed by our thoughts. If it is true that thoughts create reality, then it is imperative to create the environment that will support a successful meal plan.

In this chapter, I will help you create a strong, positive foundation that will help you achieve your health and weight loss goals on Beyond Diet.

Clear Your Mind

To truly be successful with Beyond Diet, you must clear your mind of all media information and hype. This means not believing everything you hear from so-called health and nutrition experts on TV and radio and in magazines and books. Forget all the other diets that you've tried, and remember that this plan isn't anything like those diets—it's a program that will help you lose weight while improving your overall health. If old habits keep bringing you to the same place—overweight, unhealthy, and unhappy—then you must change your approach.

Believe in What You Are Doing

For this program to be successful, you must believe in yourself. You can change your habits. You can feel great. And you can change the state of your health and weight. Forget all those times you tried different diets. This is a new day and a new approach. This time, it's about overall health.

When you begin to make any lifestyle change, you will encounter people who will try to sabotage your healthy habits in an effort to make themselves feel better. You know the people I'm talking about—the ones who say, "Oh, one won't kill you" or "Eating like that is no way to live." Well, feeling horrible each day, jeopardizing your health by carrying excess weight, not being able to keep up with your children or grandchildren, and avoiding certain activities because of your weight is no way to live. Truly believe in your new way of life and what you are doing for yourself, and don't let anyone tell you otherwise.

Eliminate Negative Thinking

Similarly, you need to free yourself from any negative thinking. If you've thought before, "What's the use? I'll only gain it back anyway," stop right there. You're through with the dieting game. Those negative thoughts are thoughts that the old you would have had, not the new, healthier you. From this point on, replace each negative thought with a positive one. The second you find yourself thinking,"I know I'm going to fail," tell yourself, "I know I can successfully change my eating habits and my life." If you repeat this statement at least five times a day, or simply use it to replace any negative thinking, I guarantee that you will begin to feel more positive and confident about your efforts to adopt a new lifestyle.

Commit Yourself to Doing the Work

Think about your biggest accomplishment to date. What did it take for you to achieve that goal? Months of overtime making yourself eligible for a job promotion? Countless hours helping your child learn a new skill? Years of practice to become successful at a sport or hobby? Accomplishment requires a great deal of work, commitment, and dedication. Achieving your health and lifestyle goals will require work. But as you know from experience, the results are worth it.

Set Goals and Positive Affirmations

Before you start the food and lifestyle changes outlined in this manual, choose three affirmations, which essentially are statements that will help you feel your best. Repeat these statements a minimum of five times per day—not out loud, so that the next person in the Shop Rite line thinks you've lost it, but to yourself—maybe in the morning as you brush your hair, in the car as you drive to work, in the afternoon as you run errands, and at night before you go to bed. The more often, the better. These statements will make you feel so good, you'll be motivated to stick with your new eating habits.

Imagine how great you'd feel if you said affirmations like these to yourself throughout the day:

I am a confident, disciplined person and can achieve anything I want.

Eating fresh, wholesome food makes me look and feel great.

I love my life, and every day of it is a blessing.

The best way to choose your own affirmations is to choose three or more goals, and then turn them into positive statements. For example, if one of your goals is to find the time to exercise more often, then one of your positive affirmations might be, "I have enough time in my day to take care of my health." Choose three important personal goals, and create three positive affirmations for yourself. After you have chosen your affirmations, write them on an index card, and carry the card with you everywhere you go.

My index card of affirmations is in my wallet. I choose not to show it to anybody, but if I have any negative thoughts during the day, I quickly pull it out and repeat my affirmations as many times as it takes to get me out of that negative mind-set. I also repeat my affirmations first thing in the morning and last thing at night. This way, I start and end my day feeling positive and inspired!

A few other ideas:

- Make extra copies of your affirmations, and leave them in places where they will remind you to repeat them during the day (e.g., in the book you're currently reading, in a desk drawer, in the kitchen).

- Tape a copy of your affirmations to the bathroom mirror, so you can give yourself a pep talk while you brush your teeth.

- Add your affirmations to your Success Journal..

Believe me when I tell you that without positive affirmations, my own journey to health would not have been possible. This single step has helped me and thousands of Beyond Diet members achieve their weight loss and lifestyle goals.

2: Three Steps to Weight Loss

Believe it or not, weight loss success is only three steps away! It might not be a quick-and-easy fix, but I promise you that **it is possible** and that **you can do it** with the guidance presented in this manual.

To be successful with Beyond Diet, you will have to do some work. This work entails many small tasks that can essentially be grouped in three main steps: Determine your metabolism type, create your personal meal plan, and learn which healthy foods you should choose.

After you have completed these three steps, you will have all the tools you need to achieve the long-term results you desire: weight loss and optimum health for life.

Step 1: Determine Your Metabolism Type

Just as you are unique in all other respects, your body's biochemistry requires certain types and proportions of healthy proteins, carbohydrates, and fats to perform optimally. This unique makeup is called your **metabolism type.** Learning your metabolism type will help you to lose weight in a safe and healthy manner, once and for all, and achieve optimum wellness. It will also will help you achieve long-term results without the starvation and cravings that usually accompany most other diet plans. What's more, it's easy to do with the questionnaire that you will complete with your Metabolism Type Test. Take the Metabolism Type Test online at:

http://go.beyonddiet.com/MetabolismTypeTest

Although volumes have been written to explain this step, you only need to know the basics to get started:

In general, everyone is a Carb Type, a Protein Type, or a Mixed Type. Each type requires ideal amounts and varieties of healthy proteins, carbohydrates, and fats (which will be explained in the Chapter on Meal Planning).

Requirements for the appropriate ratios and types of healthy proteins, carbohydrates, and fats exist along a fixed spectrum. The requirements for people whose biochemistries require high amounts of protein for optimal health (Protein Types) are located at one end, and those for people whose biochemistries demand high amounts of healthy carbohydrates (Carb Types) are at the other end. Mixed Types are a combination of these two types, so their requirements fall somewhere in the middle.

Medical doctors and nutrition pioneers have used metabolism typing for decades. It has helped people not only experience dramatic weight loss but also overcome severe chronic disease, obesity, and other serious disorders.

Learning your metabolism type will help you answer many common dietary mysteries that you have always wondered about:

Why can some people be successful—at least in losing weight over the short term—on popular low-carbohydrate, low-fat, or other diets while many others fail miserably on the same diets? Because success with any diet depends on the dieter's metabolism type; in other words, the same-diet-for-everyone approach simply is not effective.

How can one kind of food be so good for one person— giving energy and apparent health—but affect someone

else in a completely different way, making them tired and cranky? Because certain foods are ideal for each metabolism type. Just because a food is considered healthy in general does not mean that it's healthy for everyone.

Learning your metabolism type is essential to creating the meal plans that will work best for you. The ideal foods (and the ratios in which you should eat them) for your metabolism type will create the foundation for your personal meal plan. Internationally renowned natural health expert and advocate Joseph Mercola, D.O. (2005), uses metabolism typing with all of his patients for weight loss and to alleviate disease symptoms.

Step 2: Create Your Personal Meal Plan

Knowing your metabolism type, you will be able to tap into the wealth of resources needed to create a personal meal plan that will allow you to achieve long-term weight loss and optimum health. In the Chapter on Calories, you will estimate healthy daily calorie requirements for achieving and maintaining your ideal weight. Using your Success Journal, you will record your daily food intake and track how you feel afterward. Finally, the Chapter on Daily Meal Planning will guide you in choosing the ideal foods for your metabolism type, in the ideal proportions and serving sizes, and creating your own meal plan.

All of the resources you need in order to choose, combine, and portion your food properly are included in this manual and your bonus materials. The numerous charts show you the ideal ratios of proteins, carbohydrates, and fats for your metabolism type; which foods are the best choices for your metabolism type; and how to build a meal plan that takes all this personal information into account.

Step 3: Choose the Best Foods

The third, and maybe most important, step toward weight loss and overall health is to identify which foods to eat. To save yourself a lot of time, just follow this guideline: If it's natural—that is, it grows, or otherwise occurs, in nature—eat it; if it's artificial, don't. In other words, if a food contains ingredients that you can't pronounce or define, steer clear.

Natural foods span all the food groups and include fresh, unprocessed fruits and vegetables; unroasted tree nuts and ground nuts; whole seeds and grains; and unadulterated fats, dairy, and meat products. Foods in the artificial category include packaged foods, frozen meals, cookies and cakes, artificial sweeteners (e.g., saccharin [Sweet'N Low], aspartame [NutraSweet], and sucralose [Splenda]), hydrogenated oils (e.g., margarine and Crisco), high-fructose corn syrup, and any prepared products that contain any of these ingredients.

To understand why this distinction is important, you must understand the function of the liver. The liver is the body's largest internal organ, and it's responsible for an astonishing variety of life-sustaining and health-promoting tasks, including those that make healthy weight loss and weight management possible. Integral to countless metabolic processes, the liver supports the digestive system, controls blood sugar, and regulates fat storage. One of the liver's most important functions—and the one most crucial to weight loss—is the chemical breakdown of everything that enters your body.

It is the liver's job to distinguish between the nutrients to be absorbed and the dangerous or unnecessary substances to be filtered out of the bloodstream. But when overwhelmed with toxins (like artificial sweeteners and other chemicals that are added to packaged foods), the liver gets "clogged" and cannot effectively process nutrients and fats. If your liver cannot process the nutrients and fats that your body needs, you will gain weight and won't be able to lose it.

The liver also produces bile, a substance crucial to the detoxification of the body. Bile helps break down fats and assimilate fat-soluble vitamins. But when bile becomes overly congested with the toxins it's trying to filter out, it simply can't function properly. It becomes thick, viscous, and highly inefficient.

What qualifies as a toxin? Anything that your body does not recognize as a food source. Artificial sweeteners, for example, have zero calories because the body does not recognize them as food sources. But they still have to pass through the liver, as do other synthetic ingredients that you can't even pronounce.

Food-processing chemicals and other toxins also irritate the gastrointestinal system, which may manifest as bloating, constipation, or gas in many people. Chronic constipation may also lead to difficulty losing weight, not to mention a long list of other harmful health problems.

Toxins are stored in fat cells—that is, they are embedded in body fat. The more fat in your body, the more toxins you can store. Stored toxins cause your cells and organs to become sluggish and inefficient. Toxins also attack and destroy cells and gene structures. They create an acidic environment in the body that is vulnerable to fungi, bacteria, parasites, worms, viruses, and many other pathogens. Organs and body systems under a toxic load lose their ability to metabolize and process fat effectively.

The body stores toxins in fat tissue. In fact, toxin storage is one of the main functions of fat stores; this protective mechanism keeps toxins away from vital organs. When you ingest fewer toxins, your body will not need as much fat to store them and will quickly begin to let go of excess fat. This process leads to not only the right kind of weight loss (from fat) but also a healthy, disease-free body.

The body also stores toxins wherever it is weak. This makes the weak area even weaker and eventually can manifest in a cyst or disease. An area left diseased for too long becomes difficult to repair. To achieve an ideal weight and healthy body, it is vital to eat only clean, unprocessed food from this point forward.

3: Metabolism Types

Please complete the Metabolism Type Test on Beyond Diet to determine your metabolism type —Protein Type, Carb Type, or Mixed Type. Next, read through the description of (and special considerations for) your metabolism type in this chapter. You must understand why certain foods are ideal in order to make the best choices for your personal meal plan.

As you learn about your metabolism type in this chapter, remember that each person is unique, so some fine-tuning may be necessary as you change your eating habits. Pay close attention to your body's cues. Most people have fallen out of touch with their bodies and don't know what true health feels like. Pay close attention to the one and only source that knows what's best for you—your body!

Protein Types

Protein Types typically crave rich, fatty foods such as pizza, sausages, and salty roasted nuts. They love food, may not feel satiated after a snack, and often feel hungry, even after eating a large meal. When they have eaten too many carbohydrates, Protein Types tend to crave sugar. And once they start eating sugary foods, they want more and more and may find it difficult to stop. Sugar often causes Protein Types to feel jittery and will quickly make their energy levels drop.

Protein Types may have tried to lose weight by using extreme calorie-cutting methods, only to be unsuccessful—and feel miserable in the process. Protein Types cannot successfully lose weight by drastically decreasing calorie intake.

When Protein Types eat the wrong kind of food, they may notice energy problems—extreme fatigue or a wired "on edge" feeling. Eating often makes them feel better when they feel anxious, nervous, or shaky, but then they feel worse soon afterward. These cycles of energy ups and downs are definite signs of a mismatch between metabolism type and food consumption.

What Does a Protein Type Need?

Protein Types need a diet high in proteins and fats and low in carbohydrates. But think balance—not the Atkins Diet! Protein Types can eat various carbohydrates in the form of some grains, fruits, and vegetables, as long as they are adequately balanced with proteins and fats.

Because Protein Types metabolize food more quickly than other metabolism types (which is why they feel hungry all the time), heavier protein choices such as whole eggs, dark-meat poultry, beef, and dairy are essential for ideal meal planning. These foods have long been considered "unhealthy" because of their high fat content, but as you will learn in the Chapter on Fats, saturated fat is not the cause of disease; refined carbohydrates, processed foods, and hydrogenated oils are. Protein Types who do not eat heavy proteins with a high fat content will be hungry all day and struggle with their weight. Even worse, they will almost always feel fatigued and anxious.

"Must Dos" for Protein Types

- **Eat protein at every meal and with every snack.** Eating only carbohydrates at a meal causes blood sugar to spike and then drop quickly, which will leave a Protein Type feeling hungry, fatigued, and anxious as well as cause cravings for more carbohydrates shortly afterward. Eating protein—especially animal protein— at every meal and for snacks will help to control blood sugar levels and leave Protein Types feeling satiated and steady throughout the day. Remember to listen to your body—pay attention to which meals and snacks leave you hungry or craving more.

- **Eat small meals frequently or healthy snacks between meals.** Protein Types need to eat often; otherwise, they'll suffer from extremely low blood sugar levels. Going too long between meals (or snacks) also will create ravenous hunger, which in turn will cause overeating at the next meal—only to lead to lethargy and an uncomfortable feeling afterward.

- **Avoid refined carbohydrates.** Foods such as bread, crackers, and pastas—especially those made from wheat—can be extremely disruptive for Protein Types. Wheat breaks down into sugar faster than any other grain and causes the rapid release of large quantities of insulin. That is why sprouted whole grain bread products are the only allowable sources of bread. These products are described in the Chapter on Grains.

- **Avoid most fruits and fruit juices.** Fruits are a wonderful, healthy food, but Protein Types need to be extra careful with their fruit selections. Some fruits are quickly converted to sugar in the bloodstream and cause extreme blood sugar fluctuations. The best fruit choices for Protein Types are apples and avocados (high in fiber and low in sugar). Some people may be able to eat more of these fruits than others.

Carb Types

Carb Types tend to have weak appetites. They tend to be happy with a minimal amount of food each day and can get by on small amounts of food. Carb Types don't give food much thought until they feel hungry.

Carb Types tend to eat less often because they "have no time to eat." These goal-oriented workaholics will skip meals to do what they need to do each day. They may go for extended periods without eating, sending the metabolism into starvation mode. Decreasing the metabolic rate in this fashion can lead to weight management problems and obesity. Carb Types also are more dependent on caffeinated beverages to get them through the day than other metabolism types are. This dependency often weakens their appetites even more, compounding their nutritional problems.

Carb Types have a high tolerance for baked goods and starchy vegetables. This can be a bad thing, because they tend to overeat these carbohydrates, which can lead to unhealthy conditions such as hypoglycemia, insulin resistance, and diabetes.

What Does a Carb Type Need?

A Carb Type needs a diet composed of more carbohydrates than proteins or fats. But that doesn't mean that Carb Types don't need protein throughout the day. Lighter, low-fat proteins such as white-meat poultry and whitefish (e.g., tilapia, sea bass) are good choices. Carb Types can choose from a wide variety of carbohydrates and can eat them in larger quantities than any other type.

Although Carb Types convert carbohydrates into energy slowly (unlike Protein Types), it does not mean that they can go on carbohydrate binges. An elevated insulin response is still a concern, especially if weight loss is the goal. Insulin is a fat-storing hormone, so large quantities in the bloodstream will make losing weight quite difficult. Remember, excess of any particular food can lead to weight gain and disease, so always maintain the food portions and ratios recommended for your type (according to the Ideal Food Ratios For Each Metabolism Type chart).

Carb Types lose weight and feel well on a high-carbohydrate, low-fat diet—the opposite of what a Protein Type needs.

"Must Dos" for Carb Types

- **Choose low-fat proteins.** Incorporate a low-fat protein such as white-meat poultry or whitefish into each meal. Avoid (or eat only occasionally) high-fat proteins, which may cause lethargy, depression, or fatigue.

- **Choose dairy products carefully.** Carb Types tend to metabolize dairy poorly. The best way to learn whether dairy is a wise choice is to carefully monitor the body's reaction after consuming it with a meal. If you feel lethargic or fatigued shortly after, limit your dairy consumption.

- **Choose carbohydrates carefully.** Choose plenty of low-starch vegetables, like broccoli and salad greens, and limit consumption of high-starch foods such as bread, pasta, and grains. Eating too many grains may result in feeling sluggish, sleepy, or hungry soon after a meal containing a low-fat protein, a vegetable, and a grain. Try increasing the protein amount and decreasing the grain amount the next time you have this same meal.

- **Monitor your response to legumes.** Carb Types typically cannot easily digest the type of protein that most legumes contain. Therefore, eat legumes infrequently. As with all other foods, monitor the body's response carefully, and pay attention to its ability to combine them with certain foods. Some people can eat chicken, beans, and vegetables and feel great, but feel tired and sluggish if they eat beans, rice, and vegetables.

- **Limit the nuts and seeds.** Carb Types feel best on a low-fat diet, and nuts and seeds add too much fat to a meal. Nuts and nut butters are great protein choices for snacks, but lean animal meats are better protein choices for meals.

Mixed Types

A Mixed Type requires an equal balance of proteins, carbohydrates, and healthy fats, and including variety in the everyday meal plan is essential. Of the three metabolism types, this one is actually easiest to manage, because the food choices are greater. Some meals may resemble those for Protein Types, and some may resemble those for Carb Types; some may have features of both.

The appetite of a Mixed Type tends to vary greatly throughout the day—hungry at meals but not in between, ravenous at times and no appetite at others. Of course, these responses depend on what foods have been eaten that day. Mixed Types generally don't suffer from cravings. However, like the other types, Mixed Types who eat too much sugar or too many carbohydrates may develop strong sugar cravings.

Mixed Types must incorporate high-fat and low-fat proteins, as well as high-starch and low-starch carbohydrates, into their meal plans. As a Mixed Type, it is important to be familiar with the requirements of both types to find the perfect balance.

A Mixed Type may be more of a Protein Mixed Type or a Carb

Mixed Type—in other words, have more qualities of one type than the other. The only way to truly figure this out is by trial and error: by paying close attention to the body's responses to each meal, Mixed Types can determine which foods make them feel good and energized and which foods leave them feeling hungry, fatigued, cranky, or craving more. Finding the right balance of proteins, carbohydrates, and fats is the key to losing weight, feeling great, and achieving optimal health.

Weight Loss vs. Fat Loss

Losing weight and losing fat are not the same thing. To look and feel your best, you should lose weight specifically from body fat, not from muscle.

Studies often find that two groups of people consuming the same amount of calories but in different ratios of proteins, carbohydrates, and fats will lose different amounts of body fat and lean body mass (e.g., muscle and bone). For instance, someone who is a Protein Type but eats a 1,500-calorie diet composed of mostly carbohydrates each day most likely will not lose weight—or worse, may gain weight. On a 1,500-calorie diet of mostly protein, some carbohydrates, and healthy fats, this same person will reach his or her weight loss goal and feel great! (Discover the optimum food ratios for you in the Chapter on Daily Meal Planning.)

To lose weight from fat, you must focus on not only how many calories you consume but also the source of those calories (i.e., proteins, carbohydrates, or fats). Eating the foods that are ideal for your metabolism type greatly affects the source of your weight loss. When your hormones are in balance (because you're eating what your body requires), your body will achieve its ideal metabolic rate and will not need to hold onto excess fat stores—and as a result, weight loss will come from stored fat.

To conceptualize this situation, imagine yourself outside in freezing winter weather, dressed in a winter parka. If you entered a warm shelter, you would remove your coat because it would no longer be needed. The parka is like stored body fat: necessary under certain conditions but not others.

4: Calories

When most people think about weight loss and daily food consumption, the first word that comes to mind is calorie. In my experience, the mere mention of the word makes most people go pale, but at the same time, many people simply don't know what it means. For this reason, I would eliminate **calorie** from the English language if I could. The word is not bad in and of itself, but it is widely misunderstood!

In this chapter, I will present the facts about calories so you can be in-the-know. Then, I will clarify some common misconceptions about what calories are and what calories do so you can make healthy decisions about how and what to eat. Finally, you will use an easy equation to estimate your daily calorie requirements to lose weight or maintain it. Then you can forget about counting calories forever. (Really!)

Learn the Facts

According to **Merriam-Webster's Collegiate Dictionary** (11th edition), a **calorie** is "a unit equivalent to the large calorie expressing heat-producing or energy-producing value in food when oxidized in the body." In plain English, a **calorie** is a unit of energy that is released from the food you eat and used to power the body.

The body needs energy from food—calories—to perform many functions, the most obvious of which are exercise and other kinds of physical activity. However, the body also requires energy to function at the most basic level: to breathe, digest food, and maintain organs and organ systems.

Believe it or not, it is possible to eat too few calories! The most serious problem with low-calorie diets is that although they may bring about weight loss, they also can cause serious health problems. One common side effect of low-calorie diets is muscle breakdown, which can occur when the body doesn't receive enough calories from protein. Especially vulnerable is the heart, a muscular organ. If a person does not consume an adequate amount of calories each day, the heart muscle begins to break down, possibly leading to serious conditions such as cardiac atrophy.

Also, following low-calorie diets off and on over time can have negative consequences for overall health. Low-calorie diets typically do not supply enough energy to keep organs and systems healthy and, in effect, can lead to malnourishment. For clients who have repeatedly followed such diets, I recommend high-calorie meal plans that provide their organs with adequate fuel to repair themselves and regain health.

End the Calorie Debate

The American public has been told, time and time again, that consuming more calories than the body burns leads to weight gain. However, this statement is only partially true. In the following sections, I will clear up some common misconceptions about calories.

"A calorie is a calorie."

The old school of nutritional thinking teaches that all calories are created equal. Weight loss and weight gain are strictly a matter of "calories in, calories out": Regardless of the calorie source, you'll lose weight if you burn more calories than you eat and gain weight if you eat more calories than you burn.

This explanation seems logical enough, right? Unfortunately, it fails to account for modern research findings that the calories from proteins, carbohydrates, and fats have different effects on body metabolism—in other words, some calories really are healthier than others. To grasp this concept, a basic understanding of metabolism is helpful.

Two important metabolic reactions involve insulin and glucagon, hormones that are released during the digestion of food consumed. In general, **insulin** causes fat storage, and **glucagon** causes fat to be used for energy (rather than stored). The body needs both of these hormones so it can function properly, but when the insulin–glucagon balance is ideal, the body will actually build muscle while burning fat. Getting the proportions correct is key to achieving and maintaining a healthy weight, and eating the right foods for your unique metabolism type—regardless of the calorie content of those foods—is the best way to do that.

Certain foods affect insulin release much more than other foods. These foods are refined carbohydrates, which include white breads, sugars, most baked goods, and most processed snack foods. Consuming such foods causes insulin levels to increase quickly (giving a short, high energy boost) and then decrease quickly (leading to low energy levels and listlessness). When your body releases too much insulin, you may feel hungry soon after eating. Conversely, protein causes the release of glucagon, which can decrease hunger and control appetite.

By the way, it also is incorrect to say that all fats—or carbohydrates, or proteins—are created equal. Different fats (e.g., fish oil vs. hydrogenated oil) have vastly different effects on metabolism and health in general, as do different carbohydrates (e.g., low glycemic index vs. high glycemic index) and different proteins (animal vs. plant). The differences are highlighted throughout this manual.

As you see, making educated choices about where your

calories come from is important when you are attempting to control appetite, lose weight, or maintain a healthy weight in the long term.

"Calories don't matter."

This school of thought says that if you eat proteins, carbohydrates, and fats in certain ratios, then the number of calories is unimportant. For example, for proponents of metabolism typing, the only thing that matters is eating the ideal foods in the right proportions for your metabolism type. This approach can be effective if you eat those foods in the ideal amounts for your body; however, consuming larger amounts will cause you to maintain or gain weight rather than lose it.

If a meal plan for weight loss isn't created with calorie counts, then on what is it based? Ideally, each of us would know when to eat and when to stop eating simply by "listening" to the body's hunger and satiation cues. Unfortunately, though, most people who struggle with their weight have lost the ability to recognize when they are hungry or full and often eat when they feel stressed, bored, or pressured socially.

There is a way to account for this inability to listen to the body's cues, though. Estimate how many calories you need to consume daily (Determine Daily Calorie Requirements, later in this chapter - you can also do this on Beyond Diet) and then use the result as a tool to determine ideal serving sizes (Step 2: Determine Your Allowable Food Servings, in the Chapter on Daily Meal Planning, as well as on Beyond Diet). Then, by paying attention to your body's cues over time, you can create and adjust future meal plans accordingly.

"I can't eat that much and still lose weight."

Many people are surprised by the generous portion sizes and the amounts of food that this program recommends for healthy weight loss. But the truth is, with the right foods, you can eat sizable quantities of food and lose weight at the same time! Most dieters decrease their food intake so much when they want to lose weight that they do lose some pounds [kilos], then quickly plateau. At that point, they have no recourse but to eat even less food, which triggers starvation mode and makes losing weight and feeling good difficult, if not impossible.

Please don't be afraid to eat. If you eat the right foods, in the right amounts and proportions for your metabolism type, then you will lose weight and feel great. You must change your mind-set from "calorie counting" to "choosing the appropriate proportions and serving sizes" for your body. And whatever you do, don't be lured into the trap of counting calories, because that approach is not sustainable—or healthy—in the long term.

Determine Daily Calorie Requirements

Even though the word **calorie** is loaded with bad (and wrong) connotations, this program suggests estimating your daily calorie requirements as a means to an end. This number is used to determine the correct number of servings of each food type for each meal (Step 2: Determine Your Allowable Food Servings). That's it—no counting calories at each meal, or ever! (In fact, for my clients, I always did the calorie calculation myself and chose the appropriate meal plan without ever mentioning the word **calorie.**) Instead, you will use your **Success Journal** to record the individual servings of proteins, carbohydrates, and fats that you consume at each meal and your total servings for each day. A great way to keep track of all of these is in your online Success Journal on Beyond Diet.

How many calories are enough—that is, enough to provide

energy for your body to perform all its necessary functions and activities and bring about optimum health? Daily calorie requirements vary from person to person and depend on weight, foods consumed, sleep, stress and activity levels, age, and a long list of other factors that affect metabolism. Because of these many variables, no machine, calculator, or equation can determine the exact number of calories that a person needs daily. However, my experience indicates that the following calorie equation provides a good starting point, even if it is not the most scientific method.

Read the following instructions straight through once, then perform the easy calculation for yourself, recording your results here. You will need to refer to this information while you work through the Chapter on Daily Meal Planning. You can also use the online Caloric Calculator (located at **http://go.beyonddiet.com/CaloricCalculator**)—simply input your weight and choose your activity level, and your daily requirement will be calculated for you.

- Multiply your current weight (in pounds) by 13, 14, or 15 [weight (in kilograms) by 28.6, 30.7, or 33]—use 13 [28.6] if you have a particularly slow metabolism and do not exercise much, 14 [30.7] if you perform moderate exercise three or more times per week, and 15 [33] if you exercise vigorously more than three times per week. The result is your **daily calorie requirement for weight maintenance:**

  _____ pounds [kilos] × ___ = _____ calories per day

- For healthy weight loss, you must reduce your maintenance calorie intake by 20% (in other words, consume 80% of the maintenance amount). Simply multiply your daily calorie requirement for weight maintenance by 0.80. (**Note:** Do not reduce your calories by more than 20% in an effort to lose more weight; doing so may put your body in a starvation state, which would slow your metabolism and make weight loss even more difficult). The result is your **daily calorie requirement to achieve healthy weight loss:**

_____ calories × 0.80 = _____ calories per day

For example, consider a 180-pound [80-kg] female who does moderate weight training and walking three times per week.

Maintenance plan: 180 pounds × 14 = 2,520 calories per day

80 kilograms × 30.7 = 2,456 calories per day

Weight loss plan: 2,520 calories × 0.80 = 2,016 calories per day

2,456 calories × 0.80 = 1,965 calories per day

Her customized weight loss meal plan should provide about 2,000 calories per day.

Remember that these daily calorie requirements are only guidelines. Some people need fewer calories to lose weight, and others need more. The goal is to consume as many calories as possible while still losing fat, because the more fuel you give the body, the harder your metabolism will work, and you want to keep that metabolism cranking to see long-term weight loss. The truth is, the healthier your body is, the more food you can eat and still achieve or maintain your ideal weight. Calculate your daily calorie requirements online at BeyondDiet.com.

Frequently Asked Questions

What if my calorie requirements are above 2400 calories?

If your calorie requirement totals an amount above 2400 calories, begin on the 2400 calorie meal plan as your baseline serving amounts. Let your body dictate whether you need to add more or less to your plan. If you are experiencing hunger after the first 3 days, add 1-2 servings of protein, 1-2 servings of fat, and/or 1-2 servings of carbohydrate to your daily meal plan.

I want to gain weight. How do my calculations change?

If healthy weight gain is your goal, you will want to adjust your calorie calculations. Instead of subtracting 20% from your baseline calories, you will add 20%. For example, a very active male who wishes to gain weight, primarily in the form of muscle, would multiply his current weight by 15, multiply this number by 20%, and then add that total to the initial calorie calculation.

5: Daily Meal Planning

Now you have almost all the information and tools you need to begin to create your personal meal plan. In this chapter, you will learn the proper food ratios for your metabolism type, determine the ideal food servings for your daily calorie requirements, refine the food choices for your metabolism type, and then use all of this information to create your own personal meal plan—and be well on your way to weight loss success.

At this point, you should have already discovered whether you are a Protein Type, a Carb Type, or a Mixed Type according to the instructions in the Chapter on Metabolism Types or using the Metabolism Type Test on BeyondDiet.com; estimated your daily calorie requirements using the equation in the Chapter on Calories or the Caloric Calculator on BeyondDiet.com; and printed your Success Journal (or located it on BeyondDiet.com). We'll use the following charts in the Guides and Charts Chapter (towards the end of this manual) to create your meal plans in your Success Journal:

- Allowable Servings Chart
- Ideal Food Ratios For Each Metabolism Type Chart
- Food Choices Chart

Step 1: Identify Ideal Protein–Carbohydrate–Fat Ratios

On the Ideal Food Ratios for Each Metabolism Type chart, you see that different ratios of calories from proteins, carbohydrates (listed as Carbs on the chart), and fats are ideal for each metabolism type. Carb Types should eat approximately 20% proteins, 70% carbohydrates, and 10% fats; Mixed Types should eat approximately 40% proteins, 50% carbohydrates, and 10% fats; and Protein Types should eat approximately 45% proteins, 35% carbohydrates, and 20% fats.

For example, if you're a Mixed Type, each meal or snack (including your drink) should contain about half protein and half carbohydrates. (**Note:** The 10% fat would come from your protein source or from some added healthy oil.) Use the Allowable Servings Guide to create your own meal plans. You'll soon learn to tune in to your body's responses and learn when you have eaten the right amounts for you.

Step 2: Determine Your Allowable Food Servings

To determine your ideal food servings, refer to the Allowable Servings Guide. Locate the heading that lists your daily calorie requirements (as determined by the calorie equation given under Determine Daily Calorie Requirements, in the Chapter on Calories), then the column in that section that applies to your metabolism type. For example, a person who requires 2,000 calories a day and is a Protein Type should search first for the "2,000 calories/day" heading (bottom left section of the chart) and then for the Protein information (unshaded column under the "2,000 calories/day" heading). Starting from the top of this column, you can see that this person should have three protein servings and one carbohydrate serving for Breakfast, three protein servings and one carbohydrate serving for a Snack, and so on down the column.

Transfer your allowable servings information to a new page in your **Success Journal**.

After completing the Caloric Calculator and Metabolism Type Test on BeyondDiet.com, you can also access your Allowable

Servings: http://go.beyonddiet.com/AllowableServings. These servings will automatically be updated in your online Success Journal.

Step 3: Identify Your Ideal Foods

Eating the right kinds of food is just as important as eating the right quantities of food. Take a look at the Food Choices charts for your metabolism type (e.g., a Protein Type would use the Protein chart, and Carb Type would use the Carbohydrate chart; a Mixed Type would use the Mixed chart). These can be found in the Charts section of this manual, as well as online at http://go.beyonddiet.com/FoodChoices. The ideal foods for each type are shaded in the appropriate charts. Foods that are not highlighted in the charts should be avoided or eaten only occasionally. For example, an orange—generally thought of as a healthy food—will help balance a Carb Type but may push a Protein Type out of balance.

Because each person is unique, these charts must be considered as a starting point to find which foods are best for you. For example, I always test as a Protein Type but feel pretty good eating cucumbers and carrots—two foods that most Protein Types typically should avoid. When I feel lethargic soon after eating or hungry an hour later, I know I've eaten a food that isn't good for me (or that my meal didn't have the correct protein-to-carbohydrate ratio).

Again, these charts are only starting points to determine which foods might be best for you. Pay attention to how you feel after eating; track symptoms that might be related to the foods you eat in your Success Journal.

Step 4: Plan Your Meals

Finally, put all the pieces together to create a truly personal meal plan—one that meets the needs of your metabolism type and includes foods that you enjoy. Let's start with an example.

According to the Allowable Servings Guide, a Protein Type requires three protein servings at Breakfast. Possible options from the Protein Type chart could be

- 2 eggs and 1 slice of bacon
- 3 ounces [84 g] of meat or poultry (possibly leftovers from the night before)
- or something else from the chart

A Protein Type also requires one carbohydrate serving at Breakfast. Possible options from the Carbohydrate chart could be

- 1 medium apple
- 1 cup [180 g] of spinach (e.g., in an omelet)
- 1 cup [150 g] of cooked oatmeal
- or something else from the chart

For a Snack, a Protein Type requires three protein servings and one carbohydrate serving, which could be

- 1½ ounces [42 g] of raw almonds and 1 medium apple
- 3 oz [84 g] leftover turkey and ½ cup [75 g] each of celery and carrots
- or something else from the chart

Now plan a Breakfast using your unique information, and list these choices on a Meal Planning worksheet in your Success Journal under Breakfast. Refer to the example Meal Plans on the following page. (Although the serving sizes may not be exact for your needs, the sample meals demonstrate how to combine servings of proteins, carbohydrates, and fats together in a meal.) You can also plan your meals in your online Success Journal: http://go.beyonddiet.com/SuccessJournal

Do the same thing for your morning and afternoon Snacks. Keep in mind that snacks don't have to be the kinds of unhealthy, empty-calorie foods that people normally associate with snacking (chips, candy, and cookies). Healthy, nutritious snack alternatives like raw nuts and a fruit also have the advantage of being easily transportable. To choose your best snack options, think about your typical day and where you will be during mid-morning and mid-afternoon snack times. If you will be on the move, then your snack should be shelf-stable, easily transportable, and easy to eat with your hands. If you will have access to a refrigerator or a cooler, then your snack can be a mini meal that consists of leftovers from the day before.

The process of creating meals for Lunch and Dinner is the same as for Breakfast and Snacks, but you will add Fat servings, as indicated on the Allowable Servings Guide. Don't give in to society's urging to avoid all fats, thinking that doing so will help you lose weight faster. In fact, you must consume a substantial amount of healthy fat each day to lose weight, keep energy levels high, and feel satiated. (the Chapter on Fats addresses this topic in detail.) You can also look through the Recipe Guide and the Recipes section on BeyondDiet.com to help you cook up some healthy and delicious meals.

Plan another day or two of meals while you're at it, using your Success Journal.

Here are examples of what a daily meal plan may look like for each Metabolism Type:

Step 5: Learn More

Now that you have planned a few days' worth of Breakfasts, Snacks, Lunches, and Dinners, you are well on your way to achieving your ideal weight and optimum health! Your toolkit is almost complete.

Remember, the information listed in the Allowable Servings Guide (http://go.beyonddiet.com/AllowableServings) and Food Choices charts (http://go.beyonddiet.com/FoodChoices) are only suggestions and starting points. If you feel hungry at any time, you will need to adjust your meal plan in some way. Depending on your metabolism type, you might add a bit more protein, carbohydrate, or fat to a meal (to adjust the protein–carbohydrate–fat ratio slightly) or add another Snack to your day (making sure to keep that meal balanced and appropriate for your type) until you feel satiated and energized. And if something you eat makes you feel lethargic, avoid it. Likewise, if you feel that the food on your meal plans is too much food for you to eat in one day, you can also modify accordingly. Remember that I don't want you to be hungry, but I also don't want you to spend the day feeling overly full. The portion sizes in the meal plans are designed to give you a sufficient amount of food each day to feel satiated while still burning off unwanted fat. If your lifestyle or body requires less food, modify your meal plans to suit your needs.

Continue reading the rest of the manual so you can learn how to choose the best food available, prepare it in a healthy way, and enjoy your journey toward healthy weight loss. You may want to keep your Success Journal handy as you read so that you can make notes to help guide future meal planning.

6: Organic Food

What exactly is organic food? It is food grown or raised without the use of synthetic (chemically formulated) pesticides, herbicides, fungicides, or fertilizers. Organic farming allows foods to grow in nature as they were intended.

Conventional farmers in the United States alone spray 2 billion pounds [900 million kilos] of pesticides a year on crops to compensate for poor farming practices (Chek 2004, 55). And those pesticides end up in our food supply! In this chapter, I will explain why organic foods are better for your health and should be a part of your healthy lifestyle.

The Truth About Conventional Produce

In How to Eat, Move and Be Healthy, Chek (2004) lists the following chemicals found in a conventionally grown apple, a food that most of us would consider healthy!

- Chlorpyrifos: an endocrine disruptor that impairs immune response, causes reproductive abnormalities, and damages a developing nervous system

- Captan: a carcinogen (i.e., a substance believed to be capable of causing cancer) that causes genetic and immune system damage

- Iprodione: a carcinogen

- Vinclozolin: a carcinogen and a genetic, endocrine, and reproductive disruptor that causes dermatitis

Chek also provides the results of an interesting study conducted on 110 urban and suburban children in Washington state. The study found that children who ate primarily organic foods had significantly lower exposure to organophosphorous pesticide (a nervous and immune system disruptor) than children on conventional diets. Of the children tested, only one did not demonstrate measurable pesticide levels in a urine sample; this child ate an all-organic diet. The levels measured in other children who ate mainly organic foods were below the U.S. Environmental Protection Agency's (EPA's) "safe" level, whereas those of children who ate conventional foods were above this level.

Meat, Poultry, and Eggs

The animal that becomes your meal can only be as good and as healthy as the food that it was fed (in the same way that you can only be as healthy as the food you eat: You are what you eat!). In the wild, cattle eat grass, but most commercially raised cattle are fed low-quality grains to make them fat. Because these animals are not designed to eat grains, they quickly become ill, which requires the administration of antibiotics that you ingest when you eat beef.

If this situation is not bad enough, most of the chickens and pigs in commercial "factory" farms are raised in extremely small cages (usually in their own feces) and rarely see the light of day. Furthermore, they are fed a constant supply of antibiotics and growth hormones to speed growth, keep them alive, and fend off disease (Chek 2004). This fact alone should encourage you to spend the extra money on free-range organic chicken and pork.

Understandably, the quality of an egg can be only as good as the quality of the chicken that lays it, so it is crucial to buy and eat only organic eggs. A chicken that has lived a natural life produces eggs that are extremely high in Omega-3 fats—one of the healthiest types of fat for humans. As a result, the whole egg is one of the healthiest, well-balanced natural foods for humans to consume.

Many people have developed a fear of eating whole eggs because of the cholesterol in the yolk. But the truth is cholesterol is necessary for our bodies to function. However, whole eggs from commercially raised chickens are bad for us; they are high in Omega-6 fats, which cause inflammation in the body and increase the risk of heart disease.

The Value of Going Organic

As explained in Step 3: Choose the Best Foods, anything that is toxic to the body overwhelms the liver, and an overwhelmed liver becomes clogged, which makes losing weight difficult. Pesticide residues not only clog the liver but also build up on the intestinal wall, inhibiting the absorption and digestion of nutrients from the food you eat.

Some people ask whether organic food is worth the money. To me, this question is equivalent to, "Is your health worth the money?" The most common complaint or concern about "going organic" is the expense. Organic food is more expensive for several reasons. On average, organic farmers have lower yields and higher production costs than conventional farmers because they don't use herbicides; some crops are weeded by hand, which is labor-intensive. Also, organic farmers don't receive the many agricultural subsidies and other perks available to conventional farmers. You must weigh the extra cost in the short term with the long-term health benefits of sparing your body from all the chemicals. Consider our society's current state of health: The more chemicals and toxins we are exposed to, the worse our health becomes.

Consider this issue: If your doctor told you that you had a disease that required you to pay for special medical treatment to feel good every day, would you do it? I can confidently tell you that you can do something to protect your future health, prevent illness, and lose weight at the same time: spend the extra money on organic foods. You may find that when you spend less on packaged foods, the additional amount spent on organic produce and meats won't increase your overall grocery bill significantly. In addition, you will find that organic vegetables and fruits actually taste better than conventionally farmed ones.

Simply put, purchasing organic foods is an investment in your health.

With all of that being said, I understand that sometimes finding or even affording organic food may be a bit of a challenge for some. I know, because I personally experienced this. When I first discovered that organic foods would be better for my health, I was on a very tight budget (actually, I still adhere to a tight family budget and must also apply the ideas and strategies I am sharing below).

Lucky for you and me, the principles of Beyond Diet will still be effective and result in good weight loss and health results without going completely organic. You can implement this principle slowly, as your lifestyle and budget allows.

Here is how I mastered the art of "going organic on a budget":

I stopped buying processed "non foods." Most protein shakes, "health" bars, and processed foods are actually pretty expensive and when you completely eliminate them from your grocery list, you will save hundreds of dollars. Take a good look at the price of sugar cereals, packaged cookies and cakes, and frozen TV dinners. You will see how the prices of these foods quickly add up. That same amount of money can be better spent on a week's worth of organic produce.

When I started eating reasonable portions, the food was not

that expensive. When I really took a look at how much I was eating and how much I was supposed to be eating, I was eating almost double what a reasonable, healthy portion would be for me. When I started eating the correct portions for my weight and my goals, I began eating less but still feeling satisfied. Eating less meant spending less!

I sought out the local farmer's markets. The prices were so much better, and I always got fresh food in season. If there was a particular fruit that was extremely expensive during that time, I would choose a different fruit. If the berries happen to be expensive during that season, go for the apples, pears, or bananas instead. Variety is good anyway, so choose the fruits and veggies without the expensive prices.

I transitioned my kitchen and my whole house slowly. I probably did not have a completely organic kitchen until 3 years after I began. Not ideal, but I did the best I could. Rome wasn't built in a day, and neither was my organic palace. Do the best you can—start with a few items and go from there.

Buy organic foods "selectively." The following foods have been shown to have the highest levels of pesticide residue, so they should be purchased organic whenever available:

Fruits	Vegetables
1. Peaches	1. Spinach
2. Apples	2. Bell Peppers
3. Strawberries	3. Celery
4. Nectarines	4. Potatoes
5. Pears	5. Hot Peppers
6. Cherries	
7. Raspberries	
8. Imported Grapes	

These foods tend to be lower in pesticide levels so can be purchased conventional if necessary:

Fruits	Vegetables
1. Pineapples	1. Cauliflower
2. Plantains	2. Brussels Sprouts
3. Mangoes	3. Asparagus
4. Bananas	4. Radishes
5. Watermelon	5. Broccoli
6. Plums	6. Onions
7. Kiwi Fruit	7. Okra
8. Blueberries	8. Cabbage
9. Papaya	9. Eggplant
10. Grapefruit	
11. Avocado	

Action Steps

- Begin by buying organic poultry, meat, and eggs. Most supermarkets now carry organic meats, poultry and eggs. If organic products are unavailable or difficult to obtain, then the next best choice is free-range, antibiotic- and hormone-free poultry, meat, and eggs. This way, even if the animals were not fed organic feed, at least they did not receive antibiotics and hormones.

- After you have made a regular practice of buying organic (or free-range, antibiotic- and hormone-free) meat, poultry, and eggs, start buying organic produce. Begin with the produce that tends to have the highest pesticide residues as listed above.

- Remember that your success on Beyond Diet is not dependent on going completely "organic." You can still see incredible weight loss results by transitioning to organic foods slowly. Just the single step of incorporating more fruits and vegetables and natural proteins into your meal plans is a great step in the right direction towards your weight loss goals.

7: Fats

Because fat is so important for so many bodily functions, you must consume an adequate amount of fat each day. Unfortunately, our society has developed a fear of fat. In turn, many companies have produced fat-free or low-fat products that contain high amounts of sugar or high-fructose corn syrup, both of which increase hunger and cravings for sugary foods.

Because fats are an essential part of any meal plan, it is important to recognize them as good or bad. In this chapter, you'll learn how to tell the difference.

Fats to Avoid

All fats are not created equal. The most detrimental fats are hydrogenated ones called trans-fatty acids (also called TFAs or "trans fats")—most commonly listed as hydrogenated oils or partially hydrogenated oils on food labels—and should be avoided in your diet.

Hydrogenation is a chemical hardening method commonly used to create fats that are shelf-stable and have a higher melting point than their source material. To hydrogenate a liquid vegetable oil, the oil is first washed, bleached, and deodorized and then heated to a high temperature along with a metal catalyst (nickel, zinc, or copper). Next, hydrogen gas is bubbled through the mixture. Partial hydrogenation results in a product that is semisolid at room temperature (like margarine or a salad dressing oil that doesn't separate), and full hydrogenation results in a product that is solid at room temperature (like Crisco shortening). Regardless of the ultimate result, hydrogenation completely alters the liquid oil's molecular structure so that it no longer resembles a natural fat; in fact, it becomes an unhealthy trans fat. Because the body does not recognize the transformed molecule as a natural fat, it cannot process it and treats it as a toxin.

The molecular structure of a trans-fatty acid is closer to that of plastic than to that of a normal fatty acid (Chek 2004). Still, many processed foods—even some considered to be healthy—are laden with trans fats. Food manufacturers use hydrogenated oils because they have a long shelf life and are cheaper to use than the real thing, but research has shown that these fats are detrimental to your health.

Trans fats can raise levels of low-density lipoproteins (LDLs, commonly known as "bad cholesterol") and lead to clogged arteries, elevated cholesterol levels, heart disease, type 2 diabetes, and even cancer (Mercola with Droege 2003). The body has no use for trans fats and stores them in fat cells and arteries. Consuming trans fats actually causes fat cravings; these cravings continue until the body receives the essential fatty acids (EFAs)—the good fats—that it needs.

Good Fats

Good fats are derived from healthy food sources. Consuming adequate amounts of the ideal fats for your metabolism type— naturally occurring in your food, used in cooking, or taken as supplements—will fulfill your daily nutritional needs and keep you from getting hungry.

Essential Fatty Acids

The human body cannot survive without some fats— specifically, EFAs. EFAs are necessary for the healthy function of every bodily process, including

- brain and nervous system activity,
- regulation of hormones,

- function of organs and the immune system,

- cell function, and

- digestion.

Our bodies need EFAs but cannot make them on their own; therefore, we must get them from the foods we eat. The two kinds of EFAs are Omega-3 and Omega-6. Foods that are high in Omega-6 fats are grains; commercially raised meats; oils used in processed foods; and many commonly used cooking oils, including corn, safflower, and sunflower. Omega-3 fats are found in leafy green vegetables, oily fish (like salmon), walnuts, organic eggs, and naturally-raised meats.

The ideal ratio of Omega-3 to Omega-6 fats is between 1:2 and 1:4. Unfortunately, because the typical American diet is abundant in grains and cooked oils, and lacking in vegetables and healthy fish, the average Omega-6 intake is high and Omega-3 intake low. This ratio has been calculated in some people to be as high as 1:50! Clearly, we must make a conscious effort to reduce the amount of Omega-6s and increase the amount of Omega-3s that we consume to bring that ratio back toward its ideal.

Omega-3 fats are vital for the development and maintenance of the adult brain and nervous system. In The Omega Diet, Artemis Simopoulos and Jo Robinson (1998) describe a study in which mice fed a diet low in Omega-3 fats (i.e., **the most common American diet—lots of carbohydrates; packaged, processed, and fast foods; minimal fruits, vegetables, and whole foods)** led to a decreased mental performance compared with mice fed a diet with adequate Omega-3s.

Simopoulos and Robinson (1998) also state that many behavioral and mood disorders are associated with a lack of Omega-3 or an imbalance between Omega-3 and Omega-6 fats in the diet. Their list of recognized disorders (Simopoulos and Robinson 1998, 16) includes but is not limited to

- asthma,
- attention-deficit/hyperactivity disorder (ADHD),
- cancer,
- depression (even among children),
- diabetes,
- heart attack,
- insulin resistance,
- obesity, and
- stroke.

While I normally like to keep supplements to a minimum and focus more on nutrients from fresh foods, fish oil supplementation may be vital if you do not consume fresh fish on a regular basis. Also, the health of our oceans—and thus the health of the fish that live in them—is not as good as it used to be. Elevated mercury levels are increasingly found in most fresh fish sold for human consumption. Incorporate one serving of fresh fish (especially wild salmon) every week or two, but avoid fish that often have elevated levels of mercury, such as tuna, shark, and swordfish. Whatever your choices, consume at least two or three servings of Omega-3 fats daily.

The Truth About Saturated Fat

Heart disease was quite rare before 1920—so rare that the electrocardiograph (which performs the test now commonly known as an electrocardiogram [ECG]), developed to diagnose coronary heart disease, was considered a waste of time and quickly rejected. Apparently, no one suffered from clogged arteries at that time. But by the mid-1950s, heart disease was the leading cause of death among Americans. Today, heart disease causes at least 40% of all deaths in the United States each year.

In "The Skinny on Fats" (2001), the well-known nutritional expert Sally Fallon states that,

> If, as we have been told, heart disease results from the consumption of saturated fats, one would expect to find a corresponding increase in animal fat in the American diet over the same amount of time as the increase in heart disease. Actually, the converse is true. During the sixty-year period from 1910–1970, the proportion of traditional animal fat in the American diet declined from 83 percent to 62 percent, and butter consumption plummeted from eighteen pounds [eight kilograms] per person each year to four pounds [about two kilograms]. During the past eighty years, the consumption of dietary cholesterol intake has increased only one percent.

If saturated fat consumption actually decreased, then what increased? During the same period, the average intake of dietary vegetable oils (in the form of margarine, shortening, and refined oils) increased by about 400%, and the consumption of sugar and processed foods increased by about 60% (Fallon 2001).

Given this data, saturated fats apparently have been falsely accused; they are not the cause of modern disease. Unfortunately, people have been led to believe otherwise, so they try to avoid any food that contains high levels of saturated fat.

Coconut oil contains primarily saturated fat but no trans fat. It is rich in lauric acid, which is known for its antiviral, antibacterial, and antifungal properties. Some medical doctors now recommend coconut oil as a healthy food oil. In the informative online newsletter **Doctor House Call**, Al Sears, M.D. (2007), states, "The saturated fat found in coconut oil is a unique fat that helps prevent heart disease, helps to build up the immune system, and does not turn into fat in your body. In fact, it helps to speed up your metabolism ... helping you to burn fat and increase your energy!" And Joseph Mercola, D.O. (2003), claims, "Coconut oil is truly the healthiest oil you can consume" and urges readers to try virgin coconut oil and "experience the health benefits for yourself."

The saturated fat in coconut oil (as well as in palm kernel oil) is of the medium-chain fatty acid (MCFA) variety. The body digests MCFAs more easily and uses them differently than other fats. MCFAs are sent directly to the liver, where they are immediately converted into energy. In other words, the body uses the fat to make energy rather than store it (Fife 2001).

Cooking with Fats

Different types of fats respond differently to heat. Each fat has a smoke point—that is, the temperature at which it begins to smoke, become discolored, and decompose (i.e., when the fatty acid content is damaged). To avoid turning a fat rancid and unhealthy, never heat it to its smoke point. Refer to the Cooking with Fats chart to choose the best fat for each type of cooking.

In general, the two best fats to use for cooking are unrefined coconut oil (for very high heat) and raw organic butter (for medium-high heat; it should not turn brown during cooking). Because they contain high levels of saturated fat, they stay chemically stable up to 375°F. Oils that are low in saturated fat and high in monounsaturated fat, such as olive oil, are best consumed raw (e.g., on salads and vegetables) or used for light sautéing over medium heat.

Although coconut oil provides a significant amount of fat and calories, it has been proven to increase the body's metabolic rate, making it easier to lose weight. This program does not limit the amount that you can use each day. This is not to say that you should eat spoonful after spoonful all day long; a reasonable amount would be 1–2 tsp [5-10 mL] three times per day for cooking. I have never had a client not lose weight because of using too much coconut oil.

I know you're going to find it difficult to believe, but butter— at least the raw organic kind—is one of the healthiest whole foods you can include in your diet. Yes, butter contains high levels of saturated fat; but remember, saturated fat is not the culprit behind weight gain and high rates of disease. Trans fats (hydrogenated oils), sugars, and processed grains are the bad guys. Like coconut oil, butter is high in lauric acid, which the body uses for energy.

Extra-virgin olive oil is another healthy oil. It is rich in antioxidants, and 1 or 2 teaspoons [5-10 mL] go a long way (on a salad or in a sauté). When buying olive oil, look for oil that is cloudy (indicating that it has not been filtered) and has a golden yellow color (which means that it was made from fully ripened olives). Extra virgin is best. And, of course, it should be organic.

Action Steps

- Clean out your cupboards of all foods and snacks that contain hydrogenated or partially hydrogenated oil. You will find it in more packaged foods than you think, including many crackers, chips, pretzels, cookies, cereal bars, ready-to-eat cereals, microwave popcorn, and low-fat and fat-free snacks.

- Change your mind-set to no longer associate snacking with chips, crackers, and popcorn. Perfect snacks can be a smaller version of a real meal, such as a hard-boiled egg, a few pieces of chicken with vegetables, chopped vegetables, fruit, nuts, or nut butters. Fresh food is always the best food.

- Only use quality fats for cooking: coconut oil, butter (raw organic), and olive oil (unfiltered, organic, extra virgin). Brands and sources are listed in the Food Shopping Guide, which can be accessed on BeyondDiet.com at: http://go.beyonddiet.com/BDShoppingGuide

- Avoid margarine and shortening, which are hydrogenated vegetable oils.

- Consume at least two to three servings daily of good-quality Omega-3 fats from fish oil, seeds (especially flaxseed), avocados, and nuts (raw organic), especially walnuts.

- Avoid roasted nuts. The roasting process causes the fats and oils to go rancid, and rancid oils increase free-radical damage in the body. (Free radicals accelerate aging.) Some people find they digest nuts best when soaked overnight in filtered water and sea salt then dried in the oven the next day at a low temperature (no more than 150°F).

- Snack on organic nut butters. Most stores carry peanut, almond, cashew, and macadamia nut butters. The ingredient list should contain one kind of nut, salt, and nothing else. Most peanut butters contain roasted peanuts, so read labels carefully.

- Incorporate whole organic eggs into your diet, with breakfast or as a snack.

- When cooking with fat, add the fat to a cold pan and increase heat gradually.

- Serve flaxseed oil, cod liver oil, or fish oil straight from the bottle, on salads, or on cooked vegetables. Refrigerate these oils to avoid rancidity.

- If you find it difficult to incorporate foods rich in Omega-3 fats into your meal plan, take an Omega-3 supplement daily. You can learn about my favorite Omega-3 supplement, and purchase it, here: http://go.beyonddiet.com/Omega3.

8: Dairy

The subject of cow's milk dairy could fill a whole book itself. As a society, we have grown up with the idea that milk and cheese should be staples in the American diet, primarily for the calcium they purportedly provide. What researchers now know is that the quality of our milk supply has drastically changed over the past century, thus changing the daily recommended requirements for dairy from three to none. Also, many Americans now suffer from lactose intolerance and thus resort to non-dairy alternatives, which often end up causing problems worse than the dairy itself.

In this chapter, I will explain the changes in our dairy supply and the possible implications of conventional dairy consumption.

The Raw Alternative

My theories and beliefs about dairy products (i.e., milk, yogurt, and cheese) surprise many people. I believe that the only dairy products humans should consume are unpasteurized and unhomogenized, from free-roaming grass-fed cattle. Although some people fear becoming ill from raw dairy, thousands of people in this country (my family included) consume it, and not only are we not becoming sick from it, we're healthier than people who consume pasteurized dairy products.

Raw dairy can be difficult to obtain. You may have to find a raw dairy co-op that would allow you to buy a share in the ownership of a cow; in most states, the law allows the consumption of raw milk from a cow that you own, just not the sale of that milk to the public (for sources, see the Food Shopping Guide, located online at: http://go.beyonddiet.com/BDShoppingGuide

From an economic perspective, raw milk is more costly to

produce (because of the extra care given to the cows), and consumers may not be willing to pay the higher price for raw milk when cheap pasteurized milk is available. This difference is equivalent to spending more money on organic food, which may be more costly to produce but is significantly more healthy than conventionally grown food.

Conventional Milk Processing

Pasteurization

In the early 1900s, milk pasteurization began for fear of tuberculosis, botulism, and a myriad of other diseases being spread through the milk supply. Whereas this concern may have been legitimate at that time, many health professionals were (and still are) against pasteurization. For example, in **The Medical Mafia** (1995), Ghislaine Lanctôt points out that the bacteria that cause typhoid and tuberculosis are not killed by the temperatures used in pasteurization (because they are not high enough), and a good number of salmonella poisoning epidemics have been traced to pasteurized milk. In fact, all of the many incidents of salmonella-contaminated milk in recent decades occurred in pasteurized milk. One Illinois outbreak of salmonella poisoning in 1985 sickened 14,000 people and resulted in at least one death (Fallon 2001).

Because it contains bacteria that protect it from pathogens, unpasteurized milk probably does not cause illness; unfortunately, it is pasteurization that kills off this beneficial bacteria. Whereas raw milk eventually turns to buttermilk or sour cream, pasteurized milk can cause serious illness when it has gone bad.

Modern milking, packaging, and distributing methods are more sanitary than they were when pasteurization was first thought to be necessary. In my opinion, pasteurization is unnecessary and harms the milk. Lanctôt (1995) states that pasteurization destroys milk's intrinsic germicidal properties as well as its healthy enzymes (most of which are necessary for proper digestion). She goes on to state that 50% of pasteurized milk's calcium is unusable—the body cannot assimilate it. It is no wonder that the United States, rated highest in the amount of milk consumed, has a higher incidence of osteoporosis than any other country.

Many people experience extreme digestive discomfort (lactose intolerance) after consuming pasteurized dairy, which also may be laden with chemicals (added to suppress odor and restore taste) and synthetic vitamin D2 (toxic and linked to heart disease) or D3 (which is difficult to absorb) (Fallon 2001). In raw milk and raw milk products, the enzymes that aid in digestion are intact—as are the vitamins (Chek 2004). Most people who have experienced sensitivity to pasteurized dairy can tolerate raw milk.

Homogenization

Homogenization is a process whereby milk is passed through a fine filter that makes the fat molecules smaller. It enables the fat molecules to bypass digestion, increases the chances of incomplete protein digestion in the small intestine, and allows some of the milk proteins to be absorbed into the bloodstream intact, which can sensitize the immune system and lead to milk allergy and intolerance (Chek 2004).

Growth Hormone and Antibiotics

Another problem with commercially produced dairy is that cows are commonly injected with growth hormones to increase milk production. Normally, a cow produces milk for about 12 weeks after giving birth. It's a strain on her organs to produce milk that quickly. During this time, she loses weight, is infertile, and is highly susceptible to diseases such as mastitis (i.e., inflammation of the udder). By injecting a cow with recombinant bovine growth hormone (rBGH), a farmer can extend milk production for another 8–12 weeks—putting the cow under additional stress to produce milk for this extended period (Chek 2004).

The administration of rBGH also increases a cow's risk of infection by 80%. If a cow gets mastitis yet is forced to continue to produce milk, pus from the udder may end up in the milk supply. If the farmer gives the cow antibiotics to treat the infection, then those antibiotics also end up in the milk.

You may wonder why the U.S. Food and Drug Administration (U.S. FDA) would approve such a horrible practice as administering rBGH to dairy cows. The FDA states, "There is no difference between milk from treated and untreated cows" (Chek 2004, 67), but the minimal research that has been done was performed by the company that produces rBGH. Of course that company would be reluctant to release any information that may be damaging to it or its product. Chek (2004) mentions one specific study conducted by this same company. He explains that all of the animals treated with rBGH got cancer—even those that ingested it orally. This study was reviewed by employees who had previously worked for the rBGH company but were working for the FDA at the time the study was conducted.

The practices of pasteurization, homogenization, and rBGH administration in the United States will continue because the dairy industry has become a big money-making business. Many farmers are not willing to spend the time, effort, or money to raise cows naturally and ensure that they roam free and eat healthy clean grass. Because the dairy industry attempts to produce as much milk as possible (to make as much profit as possible), the cows become sick and toxic, in turn necessitating the pasteurization of their milk—purportedly to protect the health of consumers.

Yogurt

What about yogurt? Yogurt can be one of the healthiest foods if it contains live cultures of acidophilus and Bifidus, which are "good" bacteria—beneficial to the colon—in large amounts. These friendly bacteria are necessary in order to produce several vitamins and for healthy digestive function. The presence of these friendly bacteria also helps in the prevention and treatment of yeast infections.

Many people who are lactose-intolerant (cannot digest milk) can consume yogurt with no negative effects. Yogurt is easier to digest than milk because the live cultures create lactase, the enzyme that lactose-intolerant people lack.

However, as with other foods, yogurt can only be as healthy as its source, and added ingredients can change it from good to bad. When purchasing yogurt, always choose an organic brand, which will be free of antibiotics and rBGH. Also, pay close attention to the sugar content. Plain yogurt will have the lowest sugar content, and fruit-added or sweetened yogurt will have the greatest amounts. Most yogurts today contain more sugar and flavorings than candy does!

Organic yogurt can be included as a carbohydrate choice. Always look for the plain varieties and ensure that it does not contain added sugar (make sure to read the ingredients for any word ending in –ose). Six ounces [168 g] of organic plain yogurt is equal to 1 carbohydrate serving. Organic Greek yogurt can also be included, but this will count as a protein choice. Two ounces [50 g] of organic Greek yogurt = 1 protein serving.

Non-Dairy Alternatives

Almond milk and/or rice milk may be good alternatives for some when dairy and soy milk are no longer an option. Unfortunately, many brands of almond milk and rice milk contain some form of unhealthy oil (like safflower oil) and high amounts of sugar. If you can find a brand that does not add sugar or oil, you may choose to use that. Your best option is to make your own though. Here is a recipe for homemade Almond Milk: http://go.beyonddiet.com/HomemadeAlmondMilk.

Coconut milk is another great alternative to dairy milk, and it has become an absolute staple in my diet. I use it in sauces, coffee and tea, and in any recipe that calls for regular cow's milk. You can purchase the canned variety at your local health food store, as long as the ingredients list consists solely of coconut and water. Unfortunately, any canned foods are going to contain chemicals that leach from the actual can. Coconut milk also comes in cartons that can be found in the refrigerated section of most grocery stores. The problem with these is they contain ingredients like carrageenan, guar gum and evaporated cane juice. As a result, I choose to make my own coconut milk using this recipe: http://go.beyonddiet.com/HomemadeCoconutMilk.

Calcium from Non-Dairy Sources

I strongly suggest most people give up dairy and dairy products. As a result, people often wonder "Where will I get my calcium from?" Yes, calcium is vital for many functions in the body, but the amount the body actually needs and can absorb is much less than most people think. The worry that a deficiency in calcium will result when excluding dairy products is completely unnecessary.

The fact is that all leafy, green vegetables and grasses are inherently high in calcium (as well as iron, magnesium, Vitamin C, and many of the B vitamins), as are celery, cauliflower, okra, onions, green beans, avocado, black beans, chickpeas, almonds, hazelnuts, and sesame seeds. You can get plenty of calcium by adding in servings of the above foods. Take into consideration that most cows only eat grass and their bodies are naturally very high in calcium. That in itself tells us a lot.

It is also important to evaluate how much calcium is really necessary to keep your bones strong and free of osteoporosis. To do so, you must understand that one of the functions calcium has in the body is to help neutralize the acid created by eating acid forming foods like sugar, coffee, soda, and artificial sweeteners. If many of these acid-forming, calcium-robbing foods are eliminated, there will be more available calcium to create and maintain strong bones and a healthy body.

Action Steps

- If you consume dairy on a regular basis, try to buy raw (unpasteurized) certified organic products.

- If you can't obtain raw dairy products, purchase the next best thing: certified organic. Although the milk may be pasteurized, homogenized, or both, it won't contain antibiotics, hormones, or pesticide residues.

- If you can't obtain or afford raw or organic dairy products, avoid dairy altogether. Most of the calcium in dairy is not absorbed by the body anyway, so dairy is not necessary for a healthy diet. Obtain calcium from other sources, such as leafy green vegetables, broccoli, sardines (with bones), and salmon.

9: Soy

Because I recommend eliminating cow's milk from the diet, most people ask me how to replace it. Most often, they ask about soy milk.

Unfortunately, many people have been led to believe that soy and soy products are wonderfoods, but I believe that soy milk is much worse than conventional cow's milk. A lot of the "health" claims made by the soy industry are simply marketing tactics to make us spend money on soy products. The little soybean is big business; retail sales increased from $0.852 billion to $3.2 billion from 1992 to 2002. To accomplish this feat, the soy industry has had to convince a lot of people that soy is good and suppress a lot of evidence to the contrary. This truth has come to anger the many vegetarians who have long used soy as a meat replacement and now suffer from a long list of reproductive difficulties or hypothyroidism (Daniel 2005).

In this chapter, I will explain why to avoid soy.

History

The soybean is an oil-rich Asian legume (bean) that grows in fuzzy green pods. Traditionally, soybean plants were grown in Asia as green manure—a crop to be plowed under to enrich the soil between crop plantings. The Chinese found that soy consumption led to digestive discomfort, bloating, and gas. Not until they came up with fermentation methods did soy begin to be used as a food for humans.

Fermented soy products such as miso, tempeh, natto, shoyu (soy sauce), and tamari are fine to eat occasionally; fermentation deactivates some of the anti-nutrients in soy that cause digestive distress and mineral loss in bones. However, the majority of soy products sold in the United States are unfermented, so the naturally occurring toxins are intact. Unfermented soy products also are processed in a way that makes their proteins impure and increases the amount of carcinogens (Daniel 2005).

Some people argue that since Asians have been eating soy for thousands of years and have an incidence of cancer far lower than Americans, small amounts of natural fermented soy in the average Asian diet (9.3–36 grams [2–4 teaspoons] of soy per day as a condiment) may well have a protective effect. Unfortunately, Americans have taken this information and applied it incorrectly to highly processed, unfermented, low-quality soy products like tofu (a single cup of which weighs 252 grams). Many Americans eat several cups of soy products daily.

Soyfoods

In the West, the soybean has been used mostly as soybean oil, which is found in most products labeled as vegetable oil, margarine, or shortening. The soy protein left over from soy oil extraction originally was fed exclusively to animals—poultry and, more recently, farmed fish. The problem is that animals can consume only so much soy before developing serious reproductive and other health problems. As a result, the soy industry started marketing these by-products of soybean oil production to people.

A product of the industrial revolution, soy gave food technologists an opportunity to develop cheap meat substitutes. The most unhealthy modern soyfood products are manufactured using high-tech processes. They include ready-made foods such as soy sausages, soy burgers, chicken-like soy patties, packaged soy milk, protein powders, energy bars, veggie burgers, low-carbohydrate pastas, and chilis, as well as countless foods containing soy protein isolate, soy protein concentrate, and texturized vegetable protein.

Soy Isoflavones

Hormonal Effects

Just about all soy products on the market contain the phytoestrogens (plant-derived estrogens) known as isoflavones (Daniel 2005). Soy isoflavones have been shown to decrease the testosterone levels of rats, monkeys, and other animals, including humans.

In adults, soy consumption may disrupt normal hormone levels, affecting the reproductive system in women (resulting in heavier menstrual flow, increased cramping, and infertility) and decreasing testosterone levels in men (which decreases libido and lowers sperm count). In fact, a Japanese old wives' tale says that women punish straying husbands by feeding them a lot of tofu!

The effects of soy are no laughing matter, especially when it comes to the health and development of infants who are fed soy formula. Infants are extremely susceptible to the effects of soy because formula constitutes most, if not all, of their diets. Figures from the Swiss Federal Health Service indicate that, on a daily basis, an infant who is fed soy formula receives an amount of estrogen equivalent to that found in three to five birth control pills (Daniel 2005)! That's a lot of estrogen for anyone, but this amount is especially dangerous for infants whose development requires the right hormones in the right place at the right time. In boys, the onset of puberty may be delayed, and pediatricians are increasingly reporting cases of emasculated boys who reach puberty with breasts and tiny penises (Daniel 2005). In girls, the onset of puberty may be accelerated, and reproductive problems may occur in adulthood.

Thyroid Effects

Soy isoflavones damage more than the reproductive system in adults and children. People who consume high amounts of soy protein each day (e.g., in soy milk and in high-protein energy bars, which contain soy isolates—the most concentrated source of soy, still containing its isoflavones and phytoestrogens) often complain of fatigue, low energy, depression, hair loss, poor skin, weight gain, and diminished sex drive—all symptoms of low thyroid function (Daniel 2005). When tested for hypothyroidism, these people almost always test positive.

Action Steps

- Discard everything in your cupboards that contains soy protein isolate, soy protein concentrate, texturized vegetable protein, or soy (or soybean) oil. Possible products include many packaged energy bars, crackers, veggie burgers, and vegetarian look-alike products.

- If you have been consuming soy for a long time, get your thyroid function checked. If you suffer from hypothyroidism, then eliminating soy from your diet may have a positive effect on your condition.

10: Grains

For several million years, humans survived on a diet of animals and plants. As hunter–gatherers, they ate whatever they could find. With the introduction of new farming practices 10,000 years ago, humans began eating sugar and starch (in the form of grains and potatoes).

Although 10,000 years sounds like a long time, it's really only a fraction of a second in evolutionary terms, and the human body and digestive system have not evolved to process and digest high amounts of carbohydrates from starch- and sugar-rich diets. Genetically speaking, humans still have the bodies of cavemen.

Carbohydrates

Most Americans eat far too many carbohydrates—in the form of bread, cereal, pasta, corn (a grain, not a vegetable), rice, potatoes, and processed cakes and snacks—with severe consequences to their health. Making matters worse, most of these carbohydrates are consumed in the form of processed foods. After 130 years of consuming highly processed grains in the form of breads, pastries, and cereals, chronic diseases such as heart disease, elevated cholesterol, and obesity are rampant among most industrialized nations.

I do not suggest that everyone should follow a low-carbohydrate diet; everyone needs a certain amount of carbohydrates. What most people haven't realized is that the body's storage capacity for carbohydrates is quite limited, and any excess is stored as fat. Therefore, it is important to remember that vegetables and fruits also contain carbohydrates and to make the appropriate carbohydrate choices for your metabolism type. For example, the ideal foods for a Protein Type may include more above-ground vegetables and few fruits, whereas a Carb Type can tolerate starchier root vegetables and grains.

Any meal or snack high in carbohydrates generates a rapid rise in blood glucose (sugar). To compensate for this increase, the pancreas secretes insulin into the bloodstream, which lowers the glucose. Insulin, though, is essentially a hormone that stores excess carbohydrate calories (as fat in the thighs, abdomen, and buttocks) in case of famine. Even worse, high insulin levels suppress two other important hormones: glucagon and human growth hormone, which regulate the burning of fat and promote muscle development, respectively. So, the insulin from excess carbohydrates promotes fat, then inhibits the body's ability to lose that fat.

The key to successful weight loss is to first find the right quantity of carbohydrates that provide enough fuel and energy for the day (but not so many that we end up storing most of it as fat), then consume the right kind of carbohydrates to feel good and satiated after a meal.

Bread

Probably the most consumed and most popular of all carbohydrates among Americans is bread. Americans consume far too much bread, and the negative effects of its consumption are manifest in poor health and excess weight. Americans also consume the wrong kinds of bread.

The only bread allowed on this program is Food for Life brand's Ezekiel 4:9 organic sprouted whole grain (SWG) products. The process of sprouting changes a grain's composition in numerous ways to make it more beneficial as a food. It increases the content of vitamins (e.g., C, B2, B5, and B6) and beta carotene dramatically, up to eightfold. Even more important—especially considering how many people suffer from indigestion—it breaks down phytic acid (a mineral blocker). Present in the bran of all grains and the coatings of nuts and seeds, phytic acid inhibits the body's absorption of calcium, magnesium, iron, copper, and zinc and can neutralize digestive enzymes, resulting in digestive disorders. Sprouting breaks down the complex sugars responsible for intestinal gas and transforms a portion of the starch into sugar. It also inactivates aflatoxins, which are toxins produced by fungus and potent carcinogens often found in grains (Chek 2004).

The whole wheat bread that the American public has been led to believe is healthy contains processed wheat, which is deficient in nutrients. Hence the extremely high prevalence among Americans of digestive disorders such as irritable bowel syndrome and constipation. Chronic constipation can lead to many potentially dangerous health disorders and also can make losing weight quite difficult. Simply replacing bread with SWG bread can radically improve your digestion and your ability to lose weight.

Note that if you are intolerant of gluten or wheat, then you also will be intolerant of Ezekiel 4:9 organic sprouted whole grain bread. Even though sprouted grains are healthy foods for most people, the Ezekiel 4:9 ingredients include wheat and other grains that contain gluten.

Glycemic Index

Because the body converts different types of carbohydrates into sugar at different rates, the glycemic index (GI) was established to indicate how quickly a food affects blood sugar levels. Foods that have a high GI cause a rapid increase in blood glucose levels, thus a rapid release of insulin, which is exactly what you don't want when trying to lose weight and maintain good health. Foods that have a low GI cause a slow increase in blood glucose levels and a slow and controlled insulin release.

As explained earlier, insulin is a fat-storing hormone, so the more you have coursing through your bloodstream, the more likely you are to gain weight. Also, high-GI foods tend to leave you feeling hungry and craving more, whereas low-GI foods make you feel satiated and free from cravings. Refer to the Glycemic Index chart to learn the GI of each carbohydrate.

Weight loss will be much easier if you **choose low-GI** **carb**ohydrates: vegetables and some (not all) fruits. Certain types of grains and beans also have a low GI. I highly recommend that you stay away from high-GI foods when weight loss and overall health are your goals.

Gluten Intolerance

Many people cannot digest gluten—a protein found in wheat and some other grains that forms the structure of bread dough—and suffer from a mild to severe gluten intolerance. Possible symptoms of gluten intolerance include:

- abdominal pain and cramping,
- bloating and flatulence,
- bone and joint pain,
- chronic diarrhea,
- emotional disturbances such as anxiety and depression,
- fatigue (especially after eating gluten-containing foods),
- infertility,
- painful skin rash, and
- weight gain or the inability to lose weight.

If you suspect that you may be intolerant to gluten, I encourage you to eliminate gluten from your diet for at least 4–6 weeks to determine whether your symptoms are alleviated. Some gluten-containing foods and ingredients to avoid include the following:

- barley
- beer
- cold cereals (some—read ingredient lists)
- couscous
- hydrolyzed vegetable protein

- oats

- pasta

- rye

- semolina

- soy sauce

- spelt

- starch and vegetable starch

- wheat

- wheat germ

Allowable gluten-free foods and ingredients include the following:

- amaranth

- arrowroot

- bean flours (e.g., garbanzo, sorghum)

- buckwheat

- corn

- millet

- quinoa

- rice

If you feel relief from any of the above-named symptoms after following a gluten-free diet for 4–6 weeks, then you may be able to maintain a healthy weight more easily without gluten. Because most individuals who are intolerant to gluten also are intolerant to dairy, lactose, or both, I encourage you to also eliminate dairy and dairy-containing products while you're on a gluten-free diet.

Eliminating Grains

Many health experts recommend that people who suffer from chronic disease (e.g., diabetes, high blood pressure, high cholesterol, or heart disease), have struggled with obesity their whole lives, or are genetically predisposed to obesity or chronic disease completely eliminate grains from their diet. Joseph Mercola, an internationally renowned natural health physician and doctor of osteopathy, says that the major culprit behind various chronic diseases and the obesity epidemic is the overconsumption of grains and sugar. His **Total Health Program** (Mercola 2005) and The No-Grain Diet (Mercola with Levy 2003) teach optimal health and weight through grain elimination.

Mercola's No-Grain Diet (which also eliminates some other foods, such as dairy and beans) has been referred to as the Paleolithic Diet or the Caveman Diet because the allowed foods are those that were available to man before the discovery of grains. It is essentially how the first humans ate 2 million years ago. Some dieticians believe the Paleolithic Diet is the only diet coded in human genes—it allows only those foods that were available during our long evolution and discards those that were not.

Foods eliminated on a grain-free diet include:

- all gluten and gluten-free grains (as well as bread, pasta, and noodles made from grains)

- corn and corn-based products

- dairy products

- legumes (e.g., string beans, kidney beans, lentils, peanuts, snow peas, and green peas)

- potatoes (white and sweet) and yams

- sugar

- Foods allowed on a grain-free diet include

- eggs

- fruits and berries

- meat, chicken, and fish

- tree nuts (except cashews)

- vegetables (especially green vegetables)

I prescribe this way of eating to clients who have a history of diabetes, high blood pressure, high cholesterol, and heart disease or who have a long history of weight gain and difficulty losing weight. The results are truly amazing. Clients have told me that within the first week, their aches and pains went away and that they felt so much lighter and more energetic throughout the day. People suffering from digestive difficulties often feel relief in just a few days.

Rice

Rice (like most other grains) is very high in calories and carbohydrates, even in small servings. Instant rice, rice bowls, and any other rice products that have added creams, sauces, or tons of sodium are not recommended, but many other types of rice (white rice, basmati rice, black rice, jasmine, wild rice) are good choices and acceptable (in moderation) on the Beyond Diet plan.

Although many people consider brown rice a health food (and

the best option for rice), it is high in phytic acid which has the ability to grab onto other important minerals in your body, like calcium, magnesium, iron and zinc. Our bodies do not have the ability to break down phytic acid (in brown rice) and eating it can lead to mineral deficiencies. Phytic acid also inhibits enzymes that we need to digest or foods, including pepsin, which we need to digest proteins. I highly suggest you keep your intake of brown rice low, 1-2 times per month at the most, and choose from white rice, basmati rice, black rice, jasmine rice and wild rice more often.

Keep in mind that the glycemic index of a food changes drastically when combined with other foods. So regardless of your rice choice, it is essential that you combine your rice (a carb) with a healthy protein and fat any and every time you eat it. A good example of a well-proportioned meal would be 1/2 cup cooked wild rice, 4 oz beef burger, and a small green salad with an extra virgin olive oil and vinegar dressing.

Action Steps

- For all of your bread needs, consume only Food for Life's Ezekiel 4:9 organic sprouted whole grain (SWG) products (e.g., original, sesame, and cinnamon raisin loaves; rolls; English muffins; and tortillas). Use this bread to make bread crumbs for meatloaf and meatball recipes.

- Accept that breakfast and lunch do not have to include toast and sandwiches. Depending on your metabolism type, eggs, fruits, and nut butters may be great options for breakfast. Salads or vegetables with poultry, fish, or other meats may be great options for lunch.

- If you experience gastrointestinal distress (gas or bloating) while following this program, you may be gluten-intolerant. Try eliminating all gluten grains for 4–6 weeks to see whether the condition improves.

- If you continue to suffer from gastrointestinal distress after eliminating gluten grains for 4–6 weeks or if you do not lose weight after 4 weeks on this program, eliminate all grains from your diet.

11: Salt

Many people follow a low-salt diet because they have been led to believe that salt and sodium are bad and unhealthy. In this chapter I will explain why this belief may only be partially true and why salt is important in the body for several functions.

Chemically, culinary salt is NaCl—sodium chloride, made up of equal amounts sodium (Na) and chloride (Cl). "Sodium is an essential nutrient that the body cannot manufacture, yet is required for life itself. Chloride is vital for optimum health, it preserves the acid–base balance in the body, aids potassium absorption, supplies the essence of digestive stomach acid, and enhances the ability of the blood to carry carbon dioxide from respiring tissues to the lungs" (Regenerative Nutrition n.d.). But the only way to receive all of the life-sustaining benefits of salt is to consume the right kind of salt: unrefined sea salt, not processed table salt.

Salt has such a bad reputation because 99% of the world's salt research has been done on commercial table salt—the only salt that most Americans know. Some of the best scientific research on the healthy properties of unrefined sea salt are written in French, German, and Portuguese; unfortunately, few American doctors have read them. So instead of suggesting that patients use unrefined sea salt, American doctors suggest avoiding salt altogether, which can be dangerous. In many parts of France, when a person visits a physician about a heart problem or high blood pressure, the first question asked may be, "What kind of salt do you use?"

Some doctors believe that a low-salt diet can cause high blood pressure. A salt-free diet can damage heart valves and negatively affect the contractibility of the heart muscles. Biochemically, cells starve without salt.

In brief, salt:

- aids in balancing blood sugar levels.

- is needed for the absorption of food particles through the intestinal tract.

- is a strong natural antihistamine.

- can help prevent muscle cramps.

- is needed to make bones strong.

- regulates and normalizes blood pressure.

- increases energy levels.

- helps regulate the metabolism.

- helps maintain proper electrolyte balance, and

- supports the immune system.

The refined white table salt typically found at the grocery store is different from unrefined sea salt, so its effects on the body are not the same. The body cannot assimilate isolated synthetic sodium chloride (from typical refined salt), which contains none of the valuable minerals and trace elements of unrefined sea salt, so the system recognizes it as a poison. Refined table salt often contains anti-caking agents, some of which are aluminum based. (Aluminum is linked with heavy metal toxicity and possibly even Alzheimer's disease.) One such example is sodium silicoaluminate, which is thought to be associated with kidney problems and mineral malabsorption. Sodium acetate, a preservative, may cause elevated blood pressure, kidney disturbances, and water retention (Chek 2004).

I recommend that you replace refined table salt with an unrefined sea salt like AztecSeaSalt™ or Celtic Sea Salt. AztecSeaSalt™ cannot be found in stores, but it can be purchased online at http://go.beyonddiet.com/AztecSeaSalt. Celtic Sea Salt can be found in most health food stores. These unrefined sea salts are extremely healthy and have the exact opposite effect of refined salt in your body.

Unrefined sea salt provides sodium chloride in a form that that the body needs to function. It offers the perfect balance of minerals, nutrients, and sodium chloride that the body needs for optimum health. Your body can recognize and absorb these essential nutrients efficiently. According to Regenerative Nutrition, over 80 trace minerals found in the naturally filtered salt water used to create unrefined sea salt give it its vital grayish color, and its slight moistness keeps the salt and minerals in a form that the body can assimilate.

Even heart patients and people with high blood pressure can use unrefined sea salt. It has been found that the sodium in this healthy form of salt is the actual sodium that our bodies need to function properly. Processed table salt is what's causing so many people to suffer from health problems like high blood pressure. That's why I highly recommend avoiding all refined table salt and including unrefined sea salt in your meal plans instead. If you don't salt your food, add a pinch of unrefined sea salt to each liter bottle of water you drink to maintain electrolyte and energy levels.

Action Steps

- Avoid all refined white table salt.

- Avoid all high-sodium packaged and canned foods.

- Use unprocessed, unrefined AztecSeaSalt™, Himalayan pink salt, Celtic Sea Salt, or Redmond's real salt. (Other types of sea salts may contain mercury or other toxic heavy metals.)

- Always taste food before adding salt.

12: Water

If ever there were a magic potion for weight loss, water would be it. Every good nutritional program insists that you drink a minimum of 8–10 glasses of water per day. Most people don't drink the recommended amount because they don't fully understand how important water is to maintaining good health and losing weight.

Our bodies are composed of approximately 75% water. Any variation from the natural balance causes serious disruptions in many metabolic processes that are crucial to weight loss.

- **Water helps the body metabolize stored fat.** The kidneys cannot function properly without enough water. When they are not working at full capacity, the liver must take over some of the load. The liver's function is crucial to weight loss, and if the liver has to do some of the kidneys' work, it cannot adequately do its job (metabolizing fat). As a result, the liver metabolizes less fat, more fat is stored in the body, and weight loss becomes slow or stagnates.

- **Water is crucial in ridding the body of waste.** During weight loss, the body has a lot of waste to eliminate: excess fat and stored toxins. Adequate water consumption helps the body flush out these wastes.

- **Water is a natural diuretic.** Many people retain fluid and become dependent on synthetic diuretics to lose excess water weight. Surprisingly, drinking enough water is actually the best treatment for water retention. When it doesn't get enough water, the body perceives a threat to its survival and begins to hold on to every drop of water that it can. If you give your body the amount of water that it needs, it will quickly release any retained water.

- **Water is a natural laxative.** When the body does not get enough water, it takes it from other internal sources. If the colon becomes dry, stool becomes dry and difficult to pass, resulting in constipation—possibly with gas, bloating, and painful elimination. If the body receives sufficient amounts of water, the colon will be rehydrated and proper bowel function restored.

To experience significant weight loss and optimal health, it is crucial to drink a sufficient amount of water every day. By "sufficient," I mean that you should drink half your body weight (in pounds) in ounces of water each day: (body weight, in pounds/2). For example, a 200-pound person should drink 100 ounces of water. [You should drink 3 percent of your body weight (in kilos) in liters of water each day: (body weight, in kilos, x .03). For example, a 90-kilo person should drink 2.7 liters of water.]

In addition to this baseline recommendation, I suggest that you add 8 ounces [236 mL] of water for every 8 ounces [236 mL] of caffeinated beverage consumed and another 8 ounces [236 mL] if you have exercised. Also, drink water at room temperature. Cold water will sit in your stomach until it has warmed to body temperature; only then will it move to the small intestine for absorption (Chek 2004).

Many people mistake thirst for hunger because both sensations tell the brain that the body is in need of energy. As a result, a person who is dehydrated may misinterpret this feeling and end up overeating. Several studies have been done in which people were told to drink water at the first sign or feeling of hunger. In most cases, the hunger quickly passed, and subjects lost 35–40 pounds [15-20 kilos] in less than a year (Batmanghelidj 1992). If you do not drink the recommended amounts of water for your weight and experience hunger pangs during the day, then chances are your body is thirsty. Because water is a natural appetite suppressant, drink 8 ounces [236 mL] of water at the first sign of hunger and 15 minutes before the start of every meal.

Although drinking the appropriate quantity of water is essential, it is equally important to drink high-quality water. Unfortunately, no matter where you live, tap water is contaminated with heavy metals, chlorine, and waterborne toxins. I highly recommend that you filter the drinking water in your home. (Some sources are listed under **the Food Shopping Guide,** located online at: http://go.beyonddiet.com/BDShoppingGuide.) If you buy bottled water, some of the best brands are Evian, Volvic, and Fiji.

Glass containers are best to keep stored water fresh and pure. Plastic containers can leach plastic by-products into the water, affecting taste and purity, especially if exposed to direct sunlight, so always keep bottled water in a dark, cool area. Never purchase water in smoky plastic containers, which leak estrogenic chemicals (which can disrupt hormone levels) and phthalates (which have been linked to asthma and allergies) into the water.

Ideally, you also should install shower filters or, better, a whole-house water filtration system. Your skin is a living organ, and absorbing high levels of metals and chlorine from your shower and bathwater can be dangerous.

Action Steps

- Drink half of your body weight (in pounds) in ounces of water each day. Add 8 ounces of water for each 8-ounce caffeinated beverage you drink and another 8 ounces if you have exercised that day. [Drink 3 percent of your body weight (in kilos) in liters of water each day. Add 236 ml of water for each 236 mL caffeinated beverage you drink and another 236 mL of water if you have exercised that day.]

- Drink 8 ounces of water when you feel hungry.

- Drink 8 ounces of water 15 minutes before each meal.

- If you use plastic water bottles, keep them out of the sun and away from heat.

- Install filters for your drinking water and bathing water, or invest in a whole-house water filtration system.

13: Sweeteners

I introduced some caution foods as part of the "Must Dos" for each metabolism type in the Chapter on Metabolism Types. However, most commercially available sweeteners are counterproductive to a healthy lifestyle for everyone.

Sugar

It is said that for every American who eats only 5 pounds [2.5 kilos] of sugar each year, another eats 295 pounds [134 kilos]. This statistic is hard to deny, because about 60% of the U.S. population is now overweight or obese (Chek 2004).

Part of my professional responsibility to you is to not downplay the serious damage that sugar can do to your body. I am passionate about communicating the harmful effects of sugar because I have seen clients and loved ones suffer from severe complications of type 2 diabetes, the onset of which was caused directly by their consumption of sugar and refined carbohydrates. Processed sugar (which is in cakes, cookies, processed cereals, and many other foods) can literally be considered a poison, which is anything that directly causes harm and can lead to a diseased state when you ingest it.

For starters, daily sugar consumption produces a continuous acidic condition in the body. The body combats an acidic condition by taking minerals from body tissues to buffer against the acidic environment and rectify the imbalance. For example, the body may absorb calcium from bones and teeth to protect the blood. As a result, bones weaken (resulting in osteoporosis) and teeth decay (resulting in cavities). Excess sugar eventually affects every organ in the body.

Sugar has been proven to be the cause of several diseases, including diabetes, cardiovascular disease, and cancer (Mercola

2005). When the liver has stored all the sugar that it can, the excess is returned to the blood in the form of fatty acids. These fatty acids are then stored as fat in the most inactive areas of the body: belly, buttocks, breasts, and thighs. When these areas become completely filled with fat, fatty acids are then distributed among active organs (heart, liver, and kidneys), increasing the risk of developing diabetes and disease in these organs.

It is well known and well documented that cancer cells can survive only in an acidic environment and will die in an alkaline (non-acidic) environment (Quillin 2005). Sugar keeps the body in an acidic state, and tumors are enormous sugar absorbers.

Sugar consumption causes a hormonal roller coaster of alternating high levels of insulin and blood sugar. These hormonal shifts can dramatically affect your attitude and your ability to concentrate during the day. Also, if you replace nutrient-dense foods with processed sugar, the chances of acquiring one of the following diseases or side-effects skyrockets (Chek 2004):

- atherosclerosis

- attention deficit disorder and attention-deficit/ hyperactivity disorder

- behavior problems

- cancer

- chronic fatigue syndrome

- colon cancer

- coronary heart disease

- food intolerance

- kidney disease

- liver disease

- malnutrition

- osteoporosis

- overgrowth of yeast, especially Candida albicans

- tooth decay

- violent tendencies

Even if you don't consume candy or sweets outright, once you begin to read the labels of most snacks, cereals, and drinks you consume, you will notice that it doesn't take much to consume approximately 80 grams of sugar—the equivalent of 20 teaspoons [100 mL]—in a day! When reading labels, don't be thrown off by strange words like sucrose, maltose, dextrose, glucose, and the like — any word ending in -ose is a sugar. Quite often, one product will contain five or six different types of sugar. When you add up all its many forms, sugar is frequently the greatest source of total calories.

How about fruit? Fruit contains sugar, but solely in the form of fructose, whereas processed sugar (sucrose) is made up of both glucose and fructose. By itself, fructose breaks down more slowly in the body; sugar and insulin levels remain relatively constant. In contrast, sucrose is processed extremely quickly, causing a "spike" in insulin levels—rather like a power surge followed by a rapid return to baseline levels—that is stressful for the body. Fructose puts a lot less stress on the body than sucrose, and most fruits have a low GI.

The biggest mistake people make is falling for the marketing hype from juice manufacturers. They want you to think their "fresh juice" is actually good for you. If you read the package, you'll see that many such products are made "from concentrate," which could easily be translated to mean "from syrup" (Chek 2004).

Artificial Sweeteners

Some diets encourage the use of artificial sweeteners and products sweetened with them. This program does not. Consuming artificial sweeteners will keep you craving sweetness. You'll never be able to stop your carbohydrate cravings. Worse, some research indicates that artificial sweeteners create the same insulin surge as sugar (Kirsch 2005).

Artificial sweeteners signal to your taste buds, "Sweet stuff has arrived," which is translated to the brain as, "Nutrition has arrived." When the artificial sweetener reaches the small intestine, the receptors find no nutrition and send a message back to the brain, saying, "We've been tricked. There's no nutrition here." The appestat (the part of your brain that triggers satiety) therefore signals to "keep eating … to help process all this nonfood" and keep the body functioning (Chek 2004). For this reason, many people who constantly drink diet sodas are overweight and always hungry.

If you eat foods that contain some form of artificial sweetener, add up how much you consume each day. Knowing now that artificial sweeteners are toxic to the liver, how overwhelmed do you think your liver is? Does it have the ability to work properly? If weight loss or avoiding sweets has always been a problem for you, then take particular notice of how much artificial sweetener you have been ingesting. It just may be the culprit. I have seen many people experience dramatic weight and health changes just by quitting diet soda!

Even if you don't intentionally use artificial sweeteners, you must read labels. Almost every diet or sugar-free product on the market has added artificial sweetener, as do some children's snacks and most flavored waters. Read ingredient lists, and avoid all products that contain saccharin (Sweet'N Low), aspartame (NutraSweet), and sucralose (Splenda).

Stevia: A Natural Alternative

Eliminating sugar and artificial sweeteners may be difficult if you are accustomed to sweet tastes. A wonderful natural alternative to both sugar and artificial sweeteners is an herb called stevia. Extraordinarily sweet (200–300 times sweeter than sugar), stevia also is almost free of calories, so it is perfect for people who are watching their weight. Unlike sugar, it doesn't trigger a rise in blood sugar, so you won't experience a sudden increase in insulin levels. Because insulin levels and blood sugar are not affected, you won't experience a burst of energy followed by fatigue and cravings.

Stevia also presents great advantages over saccharin and other artificial sweeteners—it isn't toxic, and it has been used safely for hundreds of years. It can be used to sweeten drinks and even in baking.

If you are addicted to sodas or other beverages sweetened with sugar or artificial sweeteners, try my Tea Juice recipe in the Recipe Guide, or view it in the Recipes section on BeyondDiet. com. After only 72 hours off of sugar and sugar-containing products, your cravings will decrease drastically.

Truvia

Truvia has gotten quite a bit of attention in the media lately because it contains Stevia (a natural and healthy alternative to artificial sweeteners) but can be found at almost any local supermarket and is much cheaper than Stevia. But there is a reason why. It is not pure and contains other ingredients.

The label on the Truvia box says Erythritol, Rebiana, and Natural Flavors.

Erythritol is a natural sugar alcohol and Rebiana comes directly from the Stevia plant, but what makes me a little reluctant to use Truvia is the "Natural Flavors." When you click on the "natural flavors" link on Truvia's website to get a better explanation of what these natural flavors really are, all it says is "Natural Flavors are used to bring out the best of our natural sweetness, like pepper or salt would be used to heighten the taste of a meal." What? What does that mean? That doesn't tell me anything or indicate exactly what these natural flavors are and whether or not it could be harmful to our health.

So I don't recommend Truvia. What I recommend is natural, 100% pure Stevia.

Xylitol

Xylitol is a naturally occurring sugar in the bark of a birch tree. It is completely natural and can be used as a sweetener instead of sugar. Xylitol still does contain some calories (approximately 2.4 calories per gram compared to 4 calories per gram of sugar). Although Xylitol is a great alternative for those who wish to decrease their sugar intake, many people have a difficult time digesting Xylitol and begin to suffer from painful gas and gastrointestinal distress. Make sure to pay attention to any side effects you may be experiencing from using Xylitol.

Note: While Xyitol is safe for humans, it can be toxic for dogs. Xylitol does not affect glucose levels in people (which is why it's a great alternative to sugar), but when dogs consume it, it can cause a dangerous surge of insulin. If you suspect that your pet has eaten any food containing Xylitol, please contact your veterinarian or Animal Poison Control Center immediately.

Erythritol

Erythritol is a "sugar alcohol" that is naturally found in a wide variety of foods including mushrooms, watermelon, pears and grapes (as well as fermented foods like sake, wine and soy sauce). It has zero calories and a glycemic index of zero. And it's widely considered the "almost sugar" by health experts and pastry chefs alike. But while erythritol does a great job at mimicking the sweet taste of sugar, it behaves quite differently in the body.

First, it is slowly and incompletely absorbed from the small intestine into blood. Then, the very small amount of erythritol that is absorbed gets converted to energy by processes that require little or no insulin. That's why erythritol won't cause a spike in blood sugar levels, which is great news for anyone who is concerned about their weight!

Honey

Honey is a wonderful and natural alternative to artificial sweeteners and sugar, but it must be RAW. Raw honey is a great immune system booster, has been found to contain anti-cancer properties, helps relieve arthritis pain and assists in relieving ailments like yeast infection and athletes foot), but they did not emphasize enough that these properties have only been found in RAW honey and not pasteurized and processed honey.

Look for honey that looks thick and cloudy and specifically says "RAW" on the label and stay away from honey that has been pasteurized or processed. As with absolutely every food, be sure to use it in moderation and pay close attention to your body's response after consuming it. I use approximately 1-2 teaspoons of raw honey each day in my tea or on Ezekiel bread toast with almond butter...one of my favorite pre-workout snacks.

Maple Syrup

Maple syrup, in 100% pure (no processing or removal of anything), can be a great sweetener. Maple syrup contains manganese and zinc, natural antioxidants which are good for your immune system, male reproductive systems and helps prevent damage to the heart. It has also been found to be a potent liver cleanser, ensuring that the liver performs well.

The only problem I have seen with those who use maple syrup is that they tend to use way too much in 1 serving. One teaspoon of maple syrup can go a long way and I've even used as little as ½ teaspoon to sweeten drinks or hot cereals like oatmeal and quinoa. Maple syrup is not usually my first choice for a sweetener, as I tend to use stevia and raw honey the most, but it is still an acceptable choice on a healthy, fat burning meal plan.

Agave Syrup

Agave syrup is neither healthy nor natural (as many people believe it to be). Dr. Ingrid Kohlstadt, an associate faculty member at Johns Hopkins School of Public Health, stated "Agave is almost all fructose, a highly processed sugar with great marketing." There may be some vendors out there who are selling the real deal, but many agave sellers are actually selling a highly processed sugar that is even worse for you than high fructose corn syrup.

Chocolate

Good news for chocoholics.

As a chocolate lover myself, I do enjoy a piece of healthy chocolate every now and then. Healthy chocolate you say? Yes you heard that right. One of the biggest problems with chocolate is the heavy processing it goes through and the added sugar.

The raw cacao bean is one of nature's most fantastic superfoods due to its mineral content and wide array of unique and varied properties. Since many of the special properties of cacao are destroyed or lost by cooking, refining, and processing, we feel that planet Earth's favorite food is still unknown to most of us. Now we get to reconnect with the power of real chocolate: raw cacao beans.

With cacao beans there is fantastic hope for chocoholics everywhere! You can turn cravings for cooked, processed, chocolate into super-nutrition with raw chocolate (cacao beans).

Cacao beans are extraordinarily nutritious!

Action Steps

- Read labels! The sugar content of any food is listed right under the carbohydrate listing. Also pay attention to where the sugar is listed in the ingredients. (The order indicates relative quantity.)

- Avoid all foods that contain artificial sweeteners, sugar, or sugar derivatives.

- Avoid all sweetened beverages, including fruit juices that are not freshly juiced.

- For all your baking and sweetening needs, stevia and raw organic honey are the best choices

14: Superfoods

What exactly are "superfoods"?

In the world of healthy nutrition, we hear the term "superfood" being used a lot, but what exactly does it mean?

A superfood is a nutrient-rich food considered to be especially beneficial for health and well-being. I like to think of superfoods as foods that give you the most bang for your buck. By eating these foods, you're getting a large list of great benefits with each bite, which is a good deal if you ask me.

So, since these foods are so powerful, we would definitely want to be sure we're including them in our daily nutrition plans.

The following three foods are what I have found to be the best of the best. You'll quickly see why.

The first superfood you need to know about is...

Raw Spirulina

If you're thinking to yourself "spirul-what?" stay with me, because spirulina is the original superfood! Its history dates back to 16th century Mexico where the Aztecs ate it to improve their health. More recently, spirulina has been used to combat malnutrition in 3rd world countries.

This spiral-shaped, blue-green algae offers some other truly remarkable health benefits.

- To start, since spirulina contains over 100 nutrients, it fortifies your body in a way that keeps your belly feeling full and satisfied, reducing hunger cravings in a completely natural way.

- It contains three times the protein of a steak, keeping

your fat-burning metabolism high and excess weight melting off your problem areas.

- Spirulina also has among the highest concentrations of antioxidants of any food, which deter DNA and cell damage and reduce your risk of diseases like cancer and heart disease.

- It's a complete source of 8 amino acids which enhance muscle growth, stimulate the production of enzymes to heal your gut and improve digestion, and balance out your hormone levels.

- Aside from fish, spirulina is one of the few natural sources of Omega-3 and Omega-6 fatty acids, which are crucial for women's health (and good for men, too).

- It works as an anti-inflammatory to reduce swelling and chronic pain.

- Spirulina contains a laundry list of powerful vitamins, minerals, and nutrients you won't find in "garden variety" vegetables. It is hands-down the best source of vitamin E

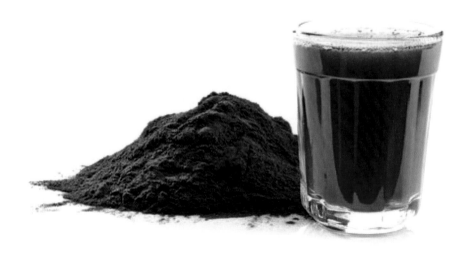

and beta carotene. It also contains extremely high levels of vitamins B1 and B2 for an all-natural energy boost, as well as calcium, potassium, niacin, and iron.

- When you take it every day, spirulina works to naturally eliminate harmful toxins from your body in just one week's time, while creating antibodies to increase your immunity and ward off illness.

- Spirulina has been shown to reduce anxiety, stress, emotional disorders, ADHD, and depression.

- AND it's been proven to reduce "bad" cholesterol.

The best part is, most people who start taking spirulina begin feeling like a better version of themselves just a few days after adding it to their diets (and who doesn't want that?) I could go on and on about the countless health benefits that simply adding a little powdered, raw spirulina to a smoothie or green drink every morning will give, but I know you don't have all day. So let's move on to superfood #2...

Wheatgrass

Since just one ounce of wheatgrass powder is nutritionally equivalent to two pounds of fresh, raw vegetables, the first "super power" of wheatgrass is that it can single-handedly make up for any nutritional deficiencies in your diet.

And it is far more common to have nutritional deficiencies in your diet than you may think. Why? Because if you buy your fruits and vegetables at the grocery store (like most people), you'll probably be surprised (and disappointed) to learn they contain far fewer vitamins than you think.

Here's why:

Due to pressure from industrial agriculture on farmers to increase crop output using the same amount of topsoil, the fruits and veggies you get from the store are grown in soil that's been stripped and depleted of its nutrients over the years. Which means, today, we only get a small fraction of the nutrients once found in the natural foods our parents and grandparents had easy access to.

The good news is, there are still some fruits and vegetables out there that are grown using traditional farming techniques, including wheatgrass. That's part of the reason wheatgrass is crucial to optimum health.

But there are even more reasons powdered wheatgrass is one of the best foods to add to your diet...

- Wheatgrass contains every single mineral known to man. (Yes... Every. Single. One.) It also contains therapeutic doses of vitamins A, B-complex, C, E, I, and K – in just one serving a day.

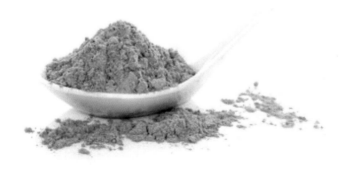

- It is made up of 70% chlorophyll, so it's literally bursting with the energy of sunlight. Chlorophyll is so valuable to our bodies because it actually helps to build blood, contains important enzymes for digestion, and acts as an antibacterial, so it naturally heals your body, inside and out.

- When taken in the right quantities and combined with certain foods, it also purifies the liver, neutralizes toxins, and eliminates harmful bacteria.

- It can help you to naturally take control of any blood sugar issues, you may have (and prevent them, if you don't); while at the same time, working to shut down your appetite, to make cravings a thing of the past.

There are so many upsides to including wheatgrass in your daily routine – it's one of the best ways to enhance your health and keep those pounds melting off your body. But there's one more superfood you need to know about if you're serious about losing weight and getting healthy. If you like chocolate as much as I do, you're going to love adding this one to your diet...

Raw Cacao

Raw cacao is not only the most delicious superfood around, though; it also contains a number of excellent nutrients that will help you improve your health and burn fat.

- Raw cacao is an amazing source of magnesium, which boosts energy, prevents osteoporosis and type 2 diabetes, and lowers blood pressure.

- It also contains super high levels of MAO inhibitors which shrink your appetite, making it easier to get from point A to point B on your weight loss journey that much faster.

- Cacao is the perfect alternative to coffee – it gives you an all-natural energy boost that lasts all day, without any downside or harsh crash.

- It makes you happy – it contains the "bliss molecule" anandamide, which improves your mood and creates a euphoric feeling – and levels out hormonal swings by boosting serotonin, the "feel good" chemical, in the brain.

- Raw cacao is good for your heart, too! It improves circulation, prevents cardiovascular disease, and lowers bad cholesterol and risk of stroke.

- Finally, raw cacao contains 4 times more antioxidants than green tea. These antioxidants prevent premature aging, keep you safe from environmental toxins, and repair damage from free radicals in your body, reducing your risk of cancer.

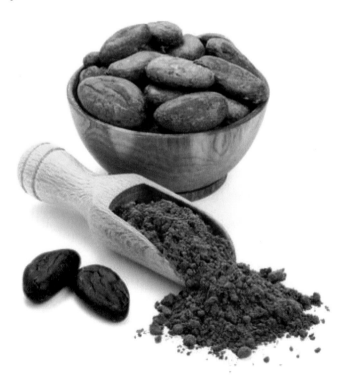

Spirulina, wheatgrass, and raw cacao are three of the most healthful and beneficial superfoods you could include in your diet. Simply adding these foods to your diet (along with the Beyond Diet eating strategies) will be a total game-changer for your health and weight loss.

But I know adding new foods to your diet can be challenging.

So if you're shaking your head and wondering how you're going to manage to include these superfoods in your diet, I get it. I've felt the same way.

That's why I started looking into other ways to include these (and many, many other) superfoods in my diet every day. I wanted to find an alternative that would provide my body with all the health benefits these superfoods provide but wouldn't require so much prep time, or involve tracking down the highest quality sources available at different health food stores or websites online.

After researching just about every possible option, I discovered an unconventional solution, called **Daily Energy** (http://go.beyonddiet.com/DailyEnergy), that provides:

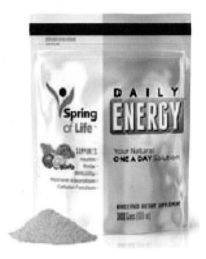

- 12 servings of fruits, greens, superfoods, mushrooms, and vegetables (a full day's worth in every serving)...

- 70 whole food ingredients, including superfoods like spirulina, wheatgrass, raw cacao (from the highest quality sources, all over the globe)...

- Countless nutrients and

minerals (many of which are not found in everyday foods)...

- Essential prebiotics, probiotics, and digestive enzymes (to improve gut health)...

- Improved weight loss results and optimum health (in just 30 seconds a day)...

- And a healthy, sustained energy boost (without any crash)...

And I'm happy to tell you that, aside from all the health benefits and enhanced weight loss properties it boasts, Daily Energy is...

A naturally sweet, 100% delicious superfood shortcut that takes just 30 seconds a day.

Not to mention, Daily Energy contains absolutely no synthetic chemicals, artificial colors, flavors, preservatives or artificial sweeteners of any kind, no GMOs, herbicides, or pesticides, no wheat, dairy, gluten, corn, lactose, sucrose, dextrose, egg, yeast, or peanuts and no animal products.

Action Steps

- Aim to include a minimum of one superfood into your eating plan every single day. You can sprinkle spirulina on your salad or add it to your favorite smoothie. It's a great way to add extra antioxidants to your already healthy meal.

Action Steps

- Make yourself a Raw Cacao Hot Chocolate first thing in the morning instead of coffee. The energy boost you get from raw cacao will last longer and won't leave you crashing mid-morning. If you're currently drinking more than 2 small coffees each day, easily lower your amount by making this delicious hot chocolate instead.

Ingredients:

1 cup coconut milk or almond milk
1 cup water
1 Tbsp cacao powder
1/2 tsp cinnamon
1 tsp vanilla extract
stevia, to taste

Directions:

Combine coconut milk (or almond milk), water, cacao, cinnamon and vanilla into a small pot and heat on low. Stir gently. Pour into 2 cups. Sweeten with a few drops of stevia to taste.

- If including these superfoods seems challenging to you on a daily basis, consider my fail proof method and take 1 scoop of Daily Energy powder (http://go.beyonddiet.com/DailyEnergy) every single day. I not only ensure that I'm getting the above 3 superfoods, I'm also getting 12 servings of fruits, greens, superfoods, mushrooms and vegetables every single day. If you or someone you love (your spouse or kids) does not enjoy eating vegetables on a daily basis, using Daily Energy is the best way to ensure you get all the benefits of veggies every single day.

15: Alcohol

Having a drink every now and then won't keep you from losing weight, but it is important to understand just how detrimental alcohol consumption is to health as well as weight-loss efforts.

You may have heard that certain types of alcohol are good for your heart and reduce cholesterol levels. Unfortunately, because of its high calorie content and toxic effects on the liver, alcohol does not support weight loss efforts. I also argue that wine consumption could negatively affect heart function more than help it.

A standard mixed alcoholic drink contains 100–250 calories, but that's only part of the problem. Most people eat more when they drink. So although you may rationalize your drink choice by thinking that you will eat less at dinner, it rarely works that way. Alcohol often makes you crave the foods you should avoid: more carbohydrates and sugar. It also may cause you to eat unhealthy foods the day after, if you feel groggy and dehydrated. Why drink something that will make it difficult for you to make healthy choices?

Alcohol is considered a carbohydrate, but your body processes it differently from other carbohydrates. Made from fermented wheat, barley, grapes, or some other carbohydrate (e.g., potatoes), alcohol contains 7 calories per gram, compared with 4 calories per gram in most carbohydrates. The human body treats alcohol as a toxin, and as a result, the liver processes alcohol calories before all others in an attempt to clean the toxins from the bloodstream. As other calories wait on line, so to speak, the body senses a rise in calories and stores many of them away in fat cells, which is exactly what you don't want when you're trying to lose weight.

In short, alcohol is the absolute worst beverage you can drink when you are trying to control the amount and types of carbohydrates in your diet. For all the reasons stated here and more, keep alcohol consumption to an absolute minimum while on a weight loss program (Kirsch 2005). After you have improved your eating habits, your body will become unable to handle as much alcohol as it did before, and you'll likely feel better overall without it. As a result, most people find that they feel best drinking no more than one glass of wine with dinner, on occasion.

I am sure you are familiar with the old saying, "It's not what you do between Christmas and New Year's, but what you do between New Year's and Christmas." An occasional indulgence every now and then won't hurt you. Just beware of the consequences. Once your body gets used to eating healthy regularly, you may experience discomfort when you indulge, such as stomach pain, bloating, or even a skin rash.

As for alcohol, there are healthier options. For instance, organic wines such as Frey are free of sulfites. Other suggestions are Skyy vodka, which is free of sulfites or unpasteurized sake. If you are still trying to lose weight, limit yourself to one or two drinks.

Action Steps

- While following this program to lose weight, drink no more than one glass per week, or, preferably, eliminate alcohol completely.

- If you drink alcohol, choose organic red wine. The rich flavor encourages you to drink slowly. Red wine also contains fewer calories and carbohydrates than other types of alcohol.

- A second-choice alcohol option is vodka on the rocks; fruit juice only adds empty sugar calories. The best brand is Chopin, which is made from potatoes, not wheat.

- After you reach your ideal weight, you can be a little more lenient, but minimize alcohol consumption to maintain a healthy weight.

16: Supplements

The diet industry has falsely led many people to believe that in order to lose weight successfully, they have to take a load of pills, eat special "diet foods" and/or drink certain "diet shakes." None of this is true, and you will see throughout this program that I make very few recommendations for supplements, and they are not required to make this program successful.

I would like to first emphasize that nothing can replace the nutritional value of real wholesome food. There may be some places in your eating plan where a supplement can prove helpful, but you always want to remember "real food is the best food."

With that being said, I do believe there are a few supplements that are worth consideration by most people and that I take myself each day. Below I have given you the supplements that I have thoroughly researched and tested and feel good recommending to my family, friends, readers and clients.

Omega-3 Supplement

I could go on and on about the long list of benefits associated with a high quality Omega-3 supplement: accelerated weight loss, increased energy, lowered risk of heart disease, and decreased risk for diabetes (just to name a few). Many people – and this may include you – are extremely deficient in Omega-3s, which can affect your ability to burn off unwanted fat. That's why I would absolutely love it if every person getting started on Beyond Diet started taking a high quality Omega-3 supplement.

Unfortunately, in my experience with certain Omega-3 products, if it smells fishy, I will most likely experience fishy burbs. All of the Omega-3s that I have recommended in the past or currently recommend do NOT cause these "fishy burps." It's just too difficult to get through my day burping up fish, no matter how much I know it's good for me.

Fishy burps are also an indication of the quality of the supplement. So if your current bottle stinks like fish, I would say that may be a first sign that it's not the best quality available.

This is the Omega-3 product I recommend using as a supplement to your Beyond Diet meal plans: http://go.beyonddiet.com/Omega3

Protein Supplements

Protein Bars

I do not use or recommend protein bars in my nutrition practice. Most bars contain soy protein which is extremely harmful to the body and can cause weight gain in many people. Many bars also contain preservatives to increase their shelf life. With wonderful, healthy "on the go" choices like raw nuts and fresh fruits, there is no need to depend on artificial food like protein bars for snacks.

Protein Powders

Many people like to use protein powders as a quick and easy form of protein. I urge you to always go for food sources of protein first (eggs, poultry, meats, fish), but when you are in the mood for a smoothie or need a quick shake in between meals, there is only 1 protein powder I feel good recommending.

The only protein powder I recommend is **BioTrust Protein Powder** (http://go.beyonddiet.com/ProteinPowder). BioTrust has formulated, what I feel, is one of the best protein powders on the market. Not only is it the best tasting protein powder I've ever had, it is made from 100% natural ingredients, with no artificial additives or toxic ingredients contained in most protein powders. This protein powder is sourced from grass fed cows that were raised naturally (not many companies can say that about their protein powders) and is sweetened with Stevia. Finally, BioTrust Protein Powder contains ProHydrolase, a digestive enzyme specifically breaks down whey protein in the body, preventing any gas or bloating while simultaneously DOUBLING your body's ability to absorb and make best use of this protein.

Greens Powder

For those who have a difficult time getting in enough servings of fruits and vegetables each day, a greens food powder is a good choice. My personal favorite is **Daily Energy** (get it here: http://go.beyonddiet.com/DailyEnergy) and I drink 1 serving each and every day. It contains 70 all natural ingredients, most of which are organic. Daily Energy is also packed with digestive enzymes, prebiotics and probiotics that all work together to improve digestion and gastrointestinal function. It contains absolutely no synthetic chemicals, artificial colors, flavors, preservatives or sweeteners of any kind; no GMOs, herbicides, or pesticides; no wheat, dairy, gluten, corn, lactose, sucrose, dextrose, egg, yeast, or peanuts; and no animal products.

Fat Burning Pills

Fat burning pills are downright dangerous and can cause severe side effects and even death, in extreme cases. Fat burning pills unnaturally elevate your heart rate and blood pressure, and can become addictive very quickly. Many people who have used fat burning pills to lose weight, almost always gain it back, sometimes more than they initially lost. Stay away from fat burning pills at all costs.

Action Steps

- Eat healthy foods that will supply you with the vitamins and nutrients you need.

- Two of the best ways to improve your health with supplements are increasing your intake of Omega-3 fatty acids (with an Omega-3 supplement) and increasing your intake of the vitamins and nutrients found in fruits and vegetables (with a greens powder).

- Avoid any and all fat burning pills!

17: Vegetarians

I do believe most people can greatly benefit from eating natural sources of animal proteins like grass fed beef, free range poultry and wild fish. Many fears vegetarians have around eating meats are the toxic and dangerous antibiotics and hormones that are added to conventional anima products. That is why I strongly recommend finding meat sources that are natural, free range, with no added antibiotics and hormones.

As much as I would love to urge everyone to include some animal products into their eating plan, being vegetarian is a personal choice and one that I do respect.

Below I have included some alternative options for vegetarians when following the program. I have seen many vegetarian readers experience great success with these modifications: losing weight, experiencing increased energy, and reversing health problems.

Depending on what type of vegetarian you are, your protein choices can include:

- eggs

- wild fish

- cottage cheese

- all varieties of raw nuts

- all varieties of raw nut butters

- all legumes*

*Vegetarians can take all of the beans and legumes listed in the "Carb Choices Chart" and make them part of their "Protein Choices Chart." This will not affect the success of the program in any way. For example, instead of having 1/2 cup of garbanzo beans be a Carb choice, it will now count as a Protein choice for that meal.

Below are some meal examples that show you how you can include a protein option (as listed above) into each and every meal.

Vegetarian breakfasts may include:

- Oatmeal with almond butter and fresh fruit
- Cottage cheese over fruit salad with walnuts sprinkled on top
- Homemade Hummus on sprouted whole grain toast

Vegetarian snacks may include:

- Baby carrots and sliced red peppers dipped in almond, peanut or walnut butter
- Raw Brazil nuts and sliced apple
- Homemade Hummus with sliced cucumbers

Vegetarian lunches and dinners may include:

- Kidney Bean and Mushroom Veggie Burger or Garbanzo Bean Burger over sauteed greens with slices of tomato on top with brown rice
- Veggie Vegetarian Chili over shredded lettuce and a sprouted grain tortilla
- Lentil and Vegetable Soup

18: Recipe Guide Overview

This guide includes some of my favorite recipes, adapted from cookbooks and online sources. Because this is not a diet in the traditional sense but a new way of eating that you want to adopt for life, it is essential that you keep your meals tasty, interesting, and creative. Eating the same foods again and again leads to boredom and abandonment. To prevent this from happening, I highly encourage you to try at least one new recipe per week that suits your meal plan. Also, be adventurous and try some foods that you have never tried before.

With all of the recipes presented here (and with any other recipe you may choose to use), adhere to all the principles taught in the manual. For example, organic ingredients are always best. Whenever possible, choose free-range, hormone- and antibiotic-free, fresh, and wild meats, poultry, eggs, and fish. Don't fear salt, but do use an unrefined sea salt or, preferably, Celtic sea salt. Oils should be cold expeller-pressed. Water should be pure and filtered. And the only breads you should consume should be made from organic sprouted whole grains (e.g., Food for Life brand's Ezekiel 4:9 products).

Also, remember that allowable food servings and portion sizes differ for each person, depending on metabolism type and the number of calories required daily. Please adjust recipe portions to suit your meal plan, as instructed in the Chapter on Daily Meal Planning, according to the Allowable Servings Guide and the Food Choices charts. For example, if you are a Carb Type allowed four 1-oz [28 g] servings of protein for dinner and a chicken recipe makes 6-oz servings (or doesn't specify a portion size), eat only 4 oz [112 g] of chicken with your meal.

Remember, fresh food is best, and the more whole and natural the food you eat, the healthier you will be—and the better you will feel. Bon appétit!

Calculating Servings for Recipes

Have a recipe you're dying to make, but not sure how to count it in your Success Journal? So many Beyond Diet members have asked how to calculate servings for recipes, so I decided to create a video explaining just that. Watch this video to learn how to calculate the carb/fat/protein servings for any recipe! I also included another (longer) recipe below as an additional example.

Kidney and Mushroom Veggie Burger

Ingredients

- 1 cup oats (dry)
- 1 14 ounce can kidney beans, drained
- ½ cup mushrooms
- ½ onion
- ½ red or yellow bell pepper
- 2 medium carrots
- 1 egg
- 2 tbsp organic ketchup (optional as it adds sugar)
- ½ tsp garlic salt

Calculation:

- 1 cup oats dry= 3 carbs
- 14 ounces kidney beans = 2 cups = 4 carbs (if you're a vegetarian, 4 proteins)
- ½ cup mushrooms = ½ carb
- ½ onion = ½ carb

- ½ pepper = about ½ cup = ½ carb
- 2 carrots = about 2 cups = 2 carb
- 1 egg = 1 protein

The ketchup doesn't count because it is such a small amount, but keep in mind that it does add sugar, so you may not even want to use it. The garlic salt is such a tiny amount (and garlic is free), so it doesn't count either.

After adding all of that up, the entire recipe makes 10.5 carbs and 1 protein (6.5 carbs and 5 proteins if a vegetarian/vegan). This should make 6 burgers, so each burger would count as 2 carbs (1 carb and 1 protein if a vegetarian/vegan).

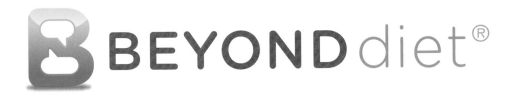

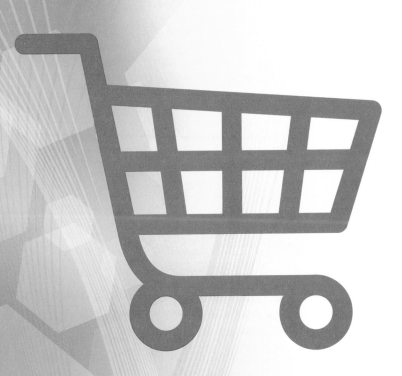

SHOPPING GUIDE

Isabel De Los Rios

Getting Started

Shopping can sometimes be overwhelming. I get it. Since it is my goal to make this way of eating simple and easy, I have created this detailed shopping guide to help you navigate the supermarket and find your essential healthy food items in a quick and cost efficient way.

This guide was truly designed to make your transition to healthy food as effortless as possible.

My goal is not only to teach you how to shop for quality food, but to save you money at the same time (and who doesn't want to save money!) It will also save you an incredible amount of time while shopping.

Throughout this guide, I mention specific product brands. I have researched these brands and personally recommend them based on their effectiveness and their fit within the program. If you cannot find these brands in person or order them online, you can make substitutions using your judgment and principles you've learned here. However, I strongly recommend you use these brands, as I have already determined that these brands deliver on their promises.

Staple Foods Shopping List

The following is a list of food items you will use most frequently. You can take this list to the store to ensure you keep your house stocked with the basics. This list should be used as a starting point for your own shopping list, based on which foods you like to eat and which you prefer to avoid. Also, meal plans or individual recipes may call for additional or more specific items.

Produce

- ORGANIC - Read more about the importance of going organic, as well as which fruits and vegetables are most important to purchase, in the Organic Food chapter of the manual

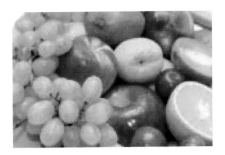 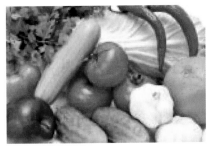

Meat/Poultry

- Grass-fed, organic beef

- Organic Chicken

- Organic Turkey

Seafood

- Wild Fish

- Shrimp, Crab and Lobster

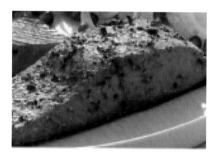 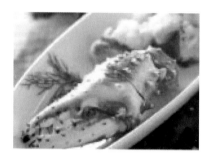

Dairy & Eggs

- Organic Eggs

- Raw (or Organic) Milk

- Raw (or Organic) Butter

- Raw (or Organic) Cheese

- Organic Plain or Organic Greek Yogurt

*For more information, refer to the Dairy chapter of the manual

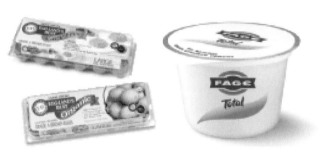 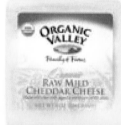

Grains

- Ezekiel Sprouted Whole Grain (SWG) Bread

- Ezekiel Cereal

- Quinoa

- Rice

*For more information, refer to the Grains chapter of the manual.

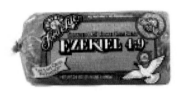 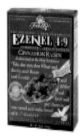 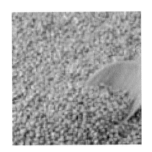

Nuts & Nut Butter

- Raw Nuts

- Raw Nut Butters - A nut butter is a spread made from crushed nuts (ex: raw almond butter).

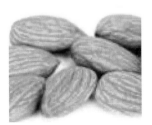 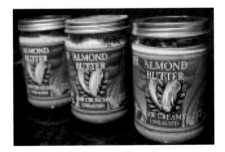

Oils (for dressings and cooking)

- Extra Virgin, Unrefined Coconut Oil

- Extra Virgin Olive Oil (EVOO)

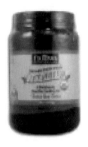 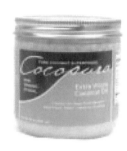 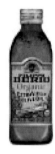

Sweeteners

- Stevia

- Raw Honey

- Pure Maple Syrup

*For more information, refer to the Sweeteners chapter of the manual.

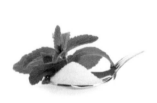 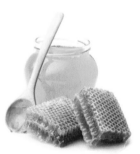 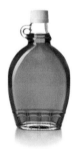

Flours

- Almond Flour

- Coconut Flour

- Spelt Flour

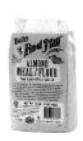 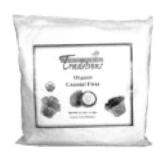 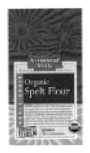

Beverages

- Coconut Milk

- Almond Milk

- Organic Tea

- Organic Coffee

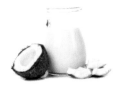 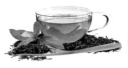 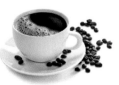

Condiments & Seasonings

- Organic Condiments (ketchup, mustard, etc.) with no added sugar

- Unrefined Sea Salt

    - AztecSeaSalt™ - Purchase online here:

        http://go.beyonddiet.com/AztecSeaSalt

- Most Herbs and Spices used in cooking are fine to continue using

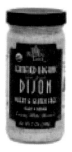 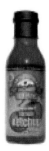 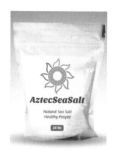

Supplements

- Daily Energy - Purchase online here:
  http://go.beyonddiet.com/DailyEnergy

- Omega-3 Supplement - Purchase online here:
  http://go.beyonddiet.com/Omega3

- BioTrust Low Carb Protein Powder - Purchase online here:
  http://go.beyonddiet.com/ProteinPowder

*For more information, refer to the Supplements chapter of the manual

Understanding The Universal Layout

Whole Foods. Wegman's. Trader Joe's. Safeway. These supermarket chains may seem very different at first glance, but they all have one major similarity - their store layout. All grocery stores, no matter how big or small, follow a universal store structure. Think about the inside of your favorite, local supermarket. When you walk through the front door, you most likely walk into the produce section first. After the produce section, you will see the seafood section. Right next door is the meat department, where you'll find chicken, beef, lamb and pork. To the left of the meat department is where you'll find dairy and eggs. Usually to the left of the dairy section you'll find fresh baked breads.

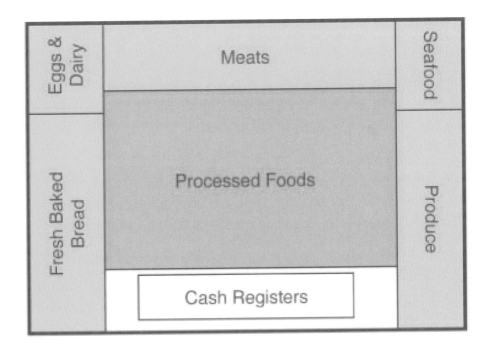

Pretty cool, huh? I bet you didn't realize that virtually all supermarkets purposely design their stores the same way.

This shopping guide follows this design as well, so that you can easily

In order to make things as easy as possible for you while you're shopping, navigate through the store from the very first page. Understanding the design of a supermarket is key to learning how to shop properly. I will elaborate on this further in the next section.

The place you should spend 90% of your time

In the above section, I mentioned the universal supermarket design. All grocery stores have a universal layout, regardless of whether it's a health food store, an organic supermarket or your neighborhood grocery store.

I am specifically referring to the foods on the perimeter aisles. All perishable items (produce, meat, seafood, dairy and fresh baked breads) are located on the "perimeters," or the edges of the store.

The perimeters are where you should spend at least 90% of your time. Why? Perishable foods are unprocessed, whole foods and, therefore, have the most nutrients and minerals.

One of the keys to achieving success with Beyond Diet is consuming delicious foods in their whole food forms. Whole foods nutritionally sustain you so that you lose weight and stay healthy at the same time.

Ironically, it's the food with the shortest shelf life that costs the most money. However, this guide will show you that healthy food does not have to leave you with a hefty grocery bill.

Throughout this guide, I will teach you how to make wise decisions in the food aisle and how to stock a healthier kitchen. You'll have complete access to the most nutritionally-balanced, budget-conscious food choices available!

I've listed the best possible options in each category in order of best choice, second best, and good choice.

Your first lesson begins in the next section - produce.

Selecting Quality Foods

Produce

Produce comes in every color of the rainbow, and it's as delicious as it is nutritious. The absolute best choice for produce is local produce. You may be surprised that my first choice wasn't organic produce. What most people do not realize is that many small local farms grow their produce without synthetic pesticides, but they cannot afford the USDA organic certification.

You may think that you can only purchase local produce at the farmer's market, but that's not true. Many supermarket chains proudly feature local produce. If you're not sure if your chain carries it, just ask.

The advantages of local produce are:

 It's the freshest produce possible;

 You are helping to support your local economy and your local farmer;

 Buying local produce means you're eating "in season;"

 You are reducing the pollution in the environment.

Organic is second best to non-synthetically pesticide grown local produce. Make sure you see the USDA Certified Organic or the USDA Organic green label (like the one to the right).

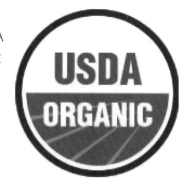

If money is no object, then by all means, purchase all of your produce in the organic section. However, if you want the healthiest options available on a budget, pay special attention to the last three paragraphs of this section.

Conventional produce is a good choice and last on the list in terms of most nutritious. Conventional produce does contain synthetic pesticides; however, not all conventional produce contain the same level of pesticides.

You can save money and reduce your exposure to pesticides by purchasing fruits and vegetables lowest in pesticides. The link below lists the dirtiest and cleanest produce. The "dirty dozen" contain 12 types of produce with very high pesticide levels. It's important that you buy these fruits and vegetables organic. The "cleanest" produce lists 20 types of produce with

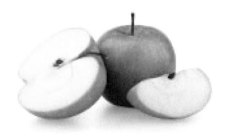

the lowest levels of pesticides - you can buy this produce conventional.

You can view a list of produce with the highest and lowest pesticide levels in the Organic Foods chapter of the manual.

Seafood

Seafood, also known as the "protein of the sea," is delicious, versatile and loaded with healthy Omega-3 fatty acids. Selecting ideal fish and seafood is crucial for optimum health benefits.

Wild caught seafood is the only seafood that I recommend. Farm raised salmon are often loaded with high levels of polychlorinated biphenyl (PCB) and are artificially colored using canthaxanthin and synthetic astaxanthin (which is not fit for human consumption).

In addition to being wild caught, you should regularly consume seafood with low mercury levels, such as salmon, cod, and herring. Fish like tuna, swordfish, and shark, although delicious, have significantly higher mercury levels - you should only eat these on occasion. I have provided a list of fish and their corresponding mercury levels at the end of this section.

My recommendation rating in this section will be based on whether seafood is fresh, frozen, or canned.

The best choice for seafood is fresh, wild caught seafood. The fish should not have a fishy odor, and the flesh should be firm to the touch. The flesh should spring back easily if you press on it. Make sure the sign on the fish explicitly says "wild caught." Ask the person behind the seafood counter to press on the flesh so you can judge the quality for yourself. If you are buying shellfish, such as shrimp, crabs, clams, mussels, octopus or squid, make sure that these are wild caught as well. If you are not sure if they are wild caught, always ask the employee behind the counter.

The second best choice for seafood is frozen seafood. Frozen seafood, in most cases, is just as healthy as fresh seafood because it is usually frozen within hours after it is caught. As with the wild seafood, make sure it clearly says "wild caught" on the packaging. Another added perk of frozen seafood is that it's usually less expensive than fresh seafood. Trader Joe's, in particular, is an affordable choice for a great variety of frozen seafood.

A good choice and even more cost efficient choice for seafood is wild caught canned seafood. Oysters, wild-caught salmon, clams, low-mercury tuna,

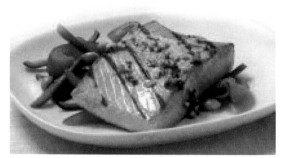

and sardines are packed with flavor, protein and Omega-3's. Canned seafood is significantly cheaper than both fresh and frozen seafood, allowing you to indulge even if you are on a strict budget. When you buy canned seafood, there are two things to look for: make sure that the seafood comes in BPA-free cans and that it is packed in pure olive oil or water. BPA (bisphenol A) is a chemical present in the lining of the can, and has been known to interfere with hormones.

Meats

When you're in the meat aisle, read the labels of the meat very carefully. The best choice for meats fits the below criteria:

- ✔ It's Organic
- ✔ It's Free-range
- ✔ It's Grass fed (pastured)
- ✔ It's Antibiotic free
- ✔ It's Hormone free

Why antibiotic and hormone free? Animals are routinely given growth hormones to make them bigger, so they produce more meat (more meat means more money). Feedlot cattle are kept in pens where they are living on top of each other. In these types of unsanitary conditions, cattle often become sick; in order to combat this, cattle are given antibiotics.

Make sure that you see all of these words on the label (please keep in mind that grass fed primarily applies to meat, not poultry, such as chicken or turkey). The meat should be fresh and should have a healthy color and hue.

Grass fed meats are usually more expensive when you purchase them in supermarkets, but cost significantly less when you purchase them directly from the farm (I will elaborate more on this in a later section).

An added benefit of grass fed meats is that they contain higher amounts of Vitamin E, Omega-3's, and a powerful fat buring compound, CLA (conjugated linoleic acid) than conventional store-bought beef. A study published in the American Journal of Clinical Nutrition proved that CLA reduces body fat without compromising muscle. CLA found in foods, such as grass fed meats and grass fed raw dairy products, is far superior to any supplement on the market.

Grass fed meat is also heart-healthy (as you can see below).

The second best choices for meats are those that are organic, free-range, and free of antibiotics and hormones.

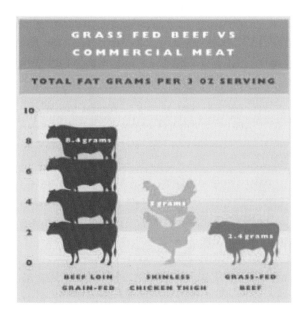

A good choice for meats, and the least expensive option for grocery bought meats, are those that are:

 Grown without the use of growth hormones (hormone free)

 Grown without the use of antibiotics (antibiotic free)

If you see the word "natural," don't be fooled. Natural does not represent livestock that have been raised without the use of hormones and antibiotics.

If you buy meats, such as bacon or cold cuts, always make sure that you purchase these items nitrate free.

Dairy/Eggs

Dairy - it's creamy, rich and yummy. And more importantly, the right dairy can be very healthy for you as well.

The best choice for dairy is raw, grass-fed dairy. Raw dairy (unpasteurized and unhomogenized) contains more Vitamins A, D, C and B vitamins than the pasteurized, homogenized store-bought version. Raw whole milk dairy also contains high levels of CLA and Omega-3 in its butterfat; in other words, this fat helps to dissolve your fat. The butterfat is also what gives the dairy a rich golden color and contributes to its rich, luscious and delicious taste! Many local farmers sell clean, nutritious, grass fed dairy (yogurt, cheese, cream, kefir, etc). If you are interested in purchasing raw dairy or would like to read about the facts behind raw dairy, pasteurization and homogenization, please visit http://realmilk.com.

The second best choice is store-bought pastured dairy that is antibiotic and hormone free (ideally unhomogenized). Brands like Organic Valley are available in many stores, and many of its dairy products (milk, cheese, heavy cream, butter) are grass fed (pastured).

A good choice for dairy is organic, antibiotic and BGH free (bovine growth hormone) that is not ultra-homogenized. Horizon is an organic brand that is sold nationwide in supermarkets.

Eggs

The criteria for buying eggs are very similar to those for buying meats. The best choice for eggs are grass fed (pastured), free range eggs, preferably from a local farm. These eggs are taken from chickens allowed to freely graze on grass and bugs (which is part of their natural diet), without being kept in cages. Not only do the eggs taste better, but the chickens are treated humanely and the eggs contain higher vitamin amounts than their store bought counterparts. You can see this in the deep rich yellow orange color of the yolk.

The second best choice is organic eggs rich in Omega-3s (ideally free-range or cage free). These chickens are fed organic feed that has higher Omega-3 levels than standard eggs.

A good choice for eggs are organic eggs (ideally free-range or cage free). These eggs come from free-range or cage free chickens (chickens who spend some time outside of a cage) that are fed natural feed.

Breads

When choosing breads, fresh with the least preservatives is always best. However, here at Beyond Diet, I want your foods to sustain your taste buds and your health. For this reason, I recommend breads that use organic sprouted grains. Why sprouted? Sprouting begins the enzymatic action that starts to break down the gluten, which makes the wheat more easily digestible and better tolerated by people with gluten sensitivities. Gluten, a protein found in wheat and grains like barley and rye, can cause digestive upsets for many people. As a matter of fact, according to a February 2003 study from the Archives of Internal Medicine, over 1.5 million Americans have celiac disease, a digestive condition aggravated by gluten.

When selecting breads, you must read the labels carefully. Look for grains in their most natural form, preferably sprouted. For example, wheat should ideally read as "sprouted wheat" on the ingredients list. If you see ingredients such as "refined wheat flour" or "unbleached enriched wheat flour," look elsewhere because these last two ingredients are forms of processed wheat.

The best choice for bread is one made from sprouted grains. A great and tasty example of sprouted whole grain (SWG) bread is Food for Life's Ezekiel 4:9 organic bread. The list of ingredients reads as follows: Organic Sprouted Wheat, Organic Sprouted Barley, Organic Sprouted Millet, Malted Barley, Organic Sprouted Lentils, Organic Sprouted Soybeans, Organic Spelt, Filtered Water, Fresh Yeast, Sea Salt.

Notice how the ingredients are simple, easy to read and understand. You should also notice how the grains listed are in their most natural form. Looking for more variety at the breakfast table than a slice of toast? Ezekiel Bread is versatile and comes in multiple varieties and flavors to fit your meal plan, such as Cinnamon Raisin Bread, English Muffins, Rolls, and Tortillas.

This bread can be found in most health food stores and supermarkets (often located in the freezer section). To find the store nearest you, visit http://www.foodforlife.com.

It's not necessary for you to buy this specific brand, but I highly recommend it. The important thing for you to do is to closely read the ingredients of any bread that you buy.

Rice Bread

If you're unable to obtain sprouted grain bread, your second best choice would be rice bread, made from rice flour. These breads are gluten and wheat free and easily digestible by the body. The first ingredient for this type of bread should be "brown rice flour." If you can't find rice bread with brown rice flour on the label; rice flour is your next best option.

Spelt Bread

A good choice, if you are not extremely intolerant to wheat or gluten, is spelt bread (spelt belongs to the wheat family and does contain gluten but is sometimes much easier to digest for people who have a difficult time digesting wheat).

You want to ensure that the first ingredient is "spelt flour."

Make sure to carefully read the label of your bread to ensure that it does NOT contain these ingredients:

- ✗ Hydrogenated Oil
- ✗ High Fructose Corn Syrup
- ✗ Bleached, enriched flour
- ✗ Wheat Gluten
- ✗ Artificial Flavor
- ✗ Sugars or Artificial Sweeteners (Aspartame or Sucralose).

No-Grain Breads

Another wonderful alternative is breads made from no grains at all. Nut flours and coconut flour are wonderful baking alternatives for anyone trying to decrease their grain intake in an effort to get their blood sugar numbers under control.

The following recipes contain no grains, wheat, or gluten, making them healthy options for those eliminating wheat and gluten from their eating plan.

Almond Flour Bread

2 ½ cups almond flour

½ tsp unrefined sea salt

½ tsp baking soda

3 cage-free, organic eggs

1 Tbsp raw honey

½ tsp apple cider vinegar

In a large bowl, combine almond flour, salt, and baking soda. In a medium bowl, whisk the eggs, then add the honey and the vinegar. Stir wet ingredients into dry. Scoop batter into a small (approximately 6" x 3"), well-greased loaf pan. Bake at 300°F for 45 to 55 minutes on bottom rack of oven until a knife comes out clean. Cool and serve.

Coconut Flour Bread

1 cup coconut flour

6 cage-free, organic eggs

½ cup coconut oil, melted

¼ cup full-fat, canned coconut milk

½ tsp unrefined sea salt

coconut oil, to grease pan

Preheat oven to 350°F. Mix dry ingredients (coconut flour and sea salt) together in a mixing bowl. Mix wet ingredients (eggs, coconut oil, coconut milk) together in a mixing bowl. Combine both wet and dry ingredients. Mix well. Mixture will look a bit dry, which is normal. Pour mixture into a bread pan greased with a little coconut oil and bake for 45 minutes. Let cool for 30 to 60 minutes.

Nut Butter Bread

1 cup raw cashew butter

4 cage-free, organic eggs (separated)

½-2 Tbsp raw honey

2 ½ tsp apple cider vinegar

¼ cup almond milk

¼ cup coconut flour

1 tsp baking soda

½ tsp unrefined sea salt

Preheat oven to 300°F. Line the bottom of a 8.5" x 4.5" glass loaf pan with parchment paper, then spread a very thin coating of coconut oil on the sides of the pan. Using an electric hand mixer, beat the cashew butter with the egg yolks, then add the honey, vinegar, and milk. Beat the egg whites in a separate bowl until peaks form. Combine the dry ingredients in another small bowl. Make sure the oven is completely preheated before adding the egg whites and the dry ingredients to the cashew butter mixture. You don't want the whites to fall and baking soda will activate once it hits the eggs and vinegar.

Pour the dry ingredients into the wet ingredients, and beat until combined. This will result in more of a wet batter than a dough. Make sure to get all of the sticky butter mixture off of the bottom of the bowl so that you don't end up with clumps. Pour the beaten egg whites into the cashew butter mixture, beating again until just combined. You don't have to be gentle with this, but don't overmix. Pour the batter into the prepared loaf pan, then immediately put it into the oven.

Bake for 45 to 50 minutes until the top is golden brown and a toothpick comes out clean. Don't be tempted to open the oven door anytime before 40 minutes, as doing so would allow steam to escape and you would not get a properly risen loaf.

Remove from the oven and let cool for 15 to 20 minutes. Use a knife to free the sides from the loaf pan, then flip the pan upside down and release the loaf onto a cooling rack. Cool right-side up for an hour before serving.

Healthy Condiments

Add on the Flavor, Not the Additives

Who doesn't like condiments? They're versatile, full of flavor and they enhance our food. While some condiments taste good, they're not necessarily good for you. This section of my guide explores condiments that elevate your taste buds and your health.

Salts

Quality salt is essential for taste and for health. Contrary to popular belief, salt is actually GOOD for you, but, not just any salt will do. Table salt and most sea salts have been processed and contain many chemical additives. These salts are stripped of their healing benefits and are not beneficial to your health.

Healthy salts are unrefined and untouched. It's important that you only purchase salt that states that it is unrefined. You can easily identify unrefined sea salt because of its unique color; natural sea salt comes in all colors ranging from grey to black. One example is AztecSeaSalt™. This salt is a light grey color because it's unprocessed. It's dried naturally by the sun and the wind. The lack of processing ensures that the trace minerals are intact. This salt supplies more than 80 trace minerals needed for optimum biological health and cell function.

AztecSeaSalt™ is a trusted brand that I highly recommend. This salt is not sold in stores, but you can purchase it here:

http://go.beyonddiet.com/AztecSeaSalt

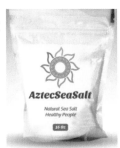

Make sure your salt does NOT contain any of the following:

✗ Sugar (added to stabilize iodine and as anti-caking chemical), or

✗ Aluminum silicate.

Sweeteners

To see how these sweeteners compare to each other, view the chart at the end of this section.

Moderation is the key to life, and when it comes to sugar, this statement is even more true. When you eat sugar, you should do so in moderation. If you do eat foods with sugar, the best choices for natural sugars are unprocessed sweeteners like raw honey, brown rice syrup, coconut sugar and pure maple syrup (Grade B). Remember, natural sugars are still sugar. Don't be fooled into thinking that because it sounds healthy, you can eat as much of it as you want. An even better alternative to natural sugars is a sugar free, healthy, natural plant-based substitute called stevia.

Brown Rice Syrup

Brown rice syrup is the sweet golden syrup by-product of cooking brown rice in water, and then evaporating most of the water. It's also wheat- and gluten-free.

Raw Honey

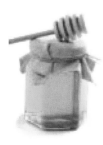

Honey, in its raw and unrefined form, contains a host of phytonutrients and enzymes that have a multitude of beneficial attributes. Refining honey uses heat, which destroys all of these enzymes and nutrients. Honey does not cause the rapid blood sugar rise and fall that white sugar does.

Pure Maple Syrup (Grade B)

Pure maple syrup is a natural sugar made from the sap of maple trees. There are two grades of pure maple syrup: Grade A and Grade B. Grade B maple syrup has a more pronounced maple flavor than Grade A. It also has a thicker consistency than grade A. Because of its rich flavor, you need less of this syrup, so you'll consume less overall sugar compared to Grade A syrup. Use both grades in moderation.

Coconut Sugar

Coconut sugar is a sugar made from the coconut flower. It is boiled down and is available in three forms: sugar blocks, soft paste, or in granular form.

Stevia

Many stevia formulations are available (e.g., liquid, powder, and powder plus inulin fiber). The liquid extract is ideal for cold beverages; the powders are ideal for baking and hot liquids. Read the packages to determine which product is right for you and the correct amounts to use in recipes. Sources include local health food stores and online.

Make sure your stevia product does NOT contain maltodextrin, dextrose, or any sugar derivative. Some stevia powders include inulin fiber. This is OK, as it's a natural fiber also found in fruits and vegetables (although some people complain that this particular fiber gives them gas and bloating). Make sure you monitor your own body's response.

Xylitol

Some people like the taste of stevia; for others, it's an acquired taste. If you don't enjoy the taste of stevia, you may want to try xylitol instead. Again, always be sure to monitor your body's response to any new food, as some people do not digest xylitol well.

The ingredients label should only list "xylitol" and no other additives.

Below is a comparison chart of the above sweeteners. All sweeteners have a Glycemic Index (GI). A GI rating measures how you blood sugar levels will respond to certain foods. The higher the number, the more drastic your blood sugar spike will be.

Sweeteners Comparison Chart	Raw Honey	Brown Rice Syrup	Coconut Palm Sugar	Pure Maple Syrup (Grade B)	Stevia (Sugar Free)	Xylitol (Sugar Free)
Glycemic Index (GI) Rating	30	25	35	54	0	7
Available in powder and liquid form					✓	✓
Is minimally processed	✓	✓	✓	✓	✓	✓
Number of calories per serving (per teaspoon)	20	23	15	17	0	10
Contains trace minerals	✓	✓	✓	✓	✓	✓
Ideal for Cold Beverages			✓		✓ *	✓
Ideal for Baking and Hot Beverages	✓	✓	✓	✓	✓ **	✓

* In liquid form

**In powder form

Oils and Fats

I recommend that you buy virgin cold-pressed, unrefined oils only (mainly olive and coconut). You should avoid all other vegetable oils (canola, soybean, etc) - the average human diet contains way too much of these ingredients. For more in-depth information about this subject, please reference the Fats chapter in the Beyond Diet manual.

Extra Virgin Olive Oil

Olive oil is a flavorful oil that is derived from - you guessed it - olives. Organic olive oil is naturally pressed and has superior taste.

For medium-heat cooking (sautéing) and use straight from the bottle (on salads and cooked foods), choose organic extra-virgin olive oil. It should be cold-pressed, cloudy (unrefined), and sold in a dark bottle.

Virgin Coconut Oil

Coconut oil has a thermogenic effect on the body, which means that it helps you to burn fat. It's also a great energy booster!

The healthy saturated fats in coconut oil have anti-microbial properties that help keep gut flora (good bacteria) in check. Coconut oil also contains high amounts of lauric acid which helps to keep your immune system strong against certain viruses, like the flu. When used topically the fatty acids in the oil deeply penetrate and moisturize your skin. A University of Kerala study reveals that virgin coconut oil speeds up your skin's collagen turnover rate. Collagen is a protein that holds the skin together, repairs broken skin, and keeps your skin wrinkle-free (added benefit, ladies). The high collagen turnover rate coconut oil provides helps to accelerate healing for burns and cuts, while the antibacterial properties of lauric acid provide a barrier against infection and germs.

Tip: For kitchen burns and cuts, always keep a small jar of virgin coconut oil near the sink.

You will receive the most benefit from coconut oil that smells and tastes of fresh coconuts.

This type of oil should be:

 Organic

 Virgin

 Cold-pressed

This type of oil should not contain any chemicals (including hexane).

Grass Fed Butter

You should also use butter for cooking, in recipes, or on top of vegetables. For high heat cooking, I recommend butter and virgin coconut oil.

Organic raw butter made from grass fed cows would be your best choice. If you are unable to find raw, organic grass fed butter, organic butter from grass fed cows is your second best choice. If either is not available, organic butter can also be used.

Make sure the ingredients on the label are:

 Organic Cream (or milk)

 Salt (I purchase unsalted and then add my own sea salt)

Grass fed butter contains vitamin K2, which is important for healthy teeth, bones and may reduce heart disease and certain cancers.

Nut Butters

Nut butter is a spreadable food made by grinding nuts into a paste. Choose nut butters (e.g., almond, walnut, cashew, or macadamia nut) made from raw - not roasted - nuts. Purchase nut butters that contain a minimal number of ingredients.

For example, an ideal almond butter ingredient label should read:

Raw (Organic) Almonds.

And that's it! Some nut butters add salt, but it is best to choose those without added salt.

Natural peanut butter is a bit more difficult to obtain in its raw state. I encourage you to try some of the other nut butter varieties (almond is my favorite!) or make your own Homemade Peanut Butter from raw peanuts. Here is a simple, delicious recipe you can try:

Homemade Peanut Butter

1 cup raw peanuts

4 Tbsp water

1-2 Tbsp of raw honey depending on taste (2 Tbsp is very sweet)

1 1/2 Tbsp coconut or extra virgin olive oil

Put all ingredients into your food processor and blend. It will become spreadable but not creamy.

Processed Foods

As a general rule, you should eat as little processed food as possible.

The main rule is to look at the product's ingredients in addition to the nutritional content in the serving column. The nutrition label can show that a product has 0g of trans fat per serving even though it is made with partially hydrogenated oils (listed in the ingredients). Make sure you read each item under the ingredients.

Avoid items with hydrogenated or partially hydrogenated oils (anything hydrogenated or partially hydrogenated is trans fat), high fructose corn syrup, artificial preservatives and flavors, artificial sweeteners (aspartame, sucralose, acesulfame potassium, saccharin, etc.), MSG, high sodium content, and high sugar content (more than 15g per serving).

When you do eat processed food, stay clear of/limit consumption of foods with the following words in the ingredients. These are hidden names for MSG.

MSG	Gelatin	Calcium Caseinate
Monosodium Glutamate	Hydrolized Vegetable Protein	Textured Protein
Monopotassium Glutamate	Hydrolized Plant Protein	Yeast Extract
Glutamate	Autolyzed Plant Protein	Yeast Food or Nutrient
Glutamic Acid	Sodium Caseinate	Autolyzed Yeast

Likewise, eliminate/reduce your consumption of processed foods containing the below ingredients. The below are hidden names for sugar. Many processed and boxed foods contain more than one of these ingredients in one product.

Dextrose	Sorbitol	Maltose
High-Fructose Corn Syrup	Corn Syrup	Invert Sugar
Malic Acid	Sucrose	Carob Powder
Maltodextrin	Glucose Syrup	Rice Malt
Diglycerides	Concentrated Fruit Juice	Levulose

Healthy Snacks

Sabatoge-Free Satisfaction

This section covers healthy snacks - yes, there is such a thing. I only recommend snacks that work with you in your weight loss efforts - not against you. These snacks are as convenient as they are tasty.

Jerky - No Slim Jims Allowed

Jerky is one of the most versatile and convenient ways to get a great source of protein. I'm not talking about the Slim Jims you buy in 7-11. Natural jerkies 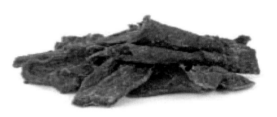 are available without nitrates or additives. They even come in an array of flavors, such as beef, buffalo, turkey and even wild salmon! The protein keeps you nice and full until your next meal.

Greek Yogurt (Full Fat) - Fat is Your Friend

Yogurt is a commonly eaten fermented food. Fermented foods are a necessity in our diet. They help keep a balance of healthy bacteria or flora (probiotics) within your gut.

Full fat Greek yogurt tastes so delicious, you may forget that it's good for you. Greek yogurt has a thick, custard-like consistency that has more protein than plain yogurt. The full fat in the yogurt keeps you fuller for longer between meals. Fage is a brand available nationwide. I recommend Fage Total, which is the full fat version of the yogurt. For a guilt-free touch of sweetness, add stevia or a tablespoon of raw honey and a handful of raw nuts for an added protein boost.

For those who prefer the taste of traditional yogurt, your best choice would be raw, grass fed yogurt. Your second best choice for healthy yogurt is organic, grass fed yogurt. If you are unable to locate one of the first two choices, a good choice is an organic, hormone and antibiotic free store bought brand, such as Stonyfield. Opt for the plain flavor, as this has the least 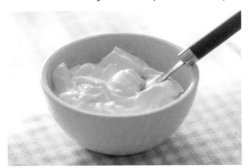 amount of sugar (you can always add your own fruit and/or natural sweetener/ sugar substitute at home).

Smoked Oysters and Sardines

Get your protein and Omega-3s in one place. Naturally smoked oysters and sardines, by Crown Prince, provide a whopping 10 grams of protein per can! Both products are packed in extra virgin olive oil for a good source of heart healthy monounsaturated fats.

Raw Nuts

Raw nuts – almonds, walnuts, cashews, etc. – are an excellent source of protein. Pair them with fresh fruit or veggies for a healthy, balanced snack.

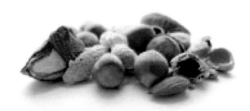

Raw Cheese

Raw milk cheese is a great source of CLA, a fat-fighting compound that occurs naturally in this food. It is also a good source of protein. Pair this treat with a low sugar fruit, like an apple, for a mid-afternoon delight.

Beverages

Although water is an ideal beverage, let's face it - every now and then you want something different. There are more and more healthy beverages being released on the market each day. Below is a brand that I recommend.

Honest Teas

Honest Teas is a NY based beverage company that was launched in 1998. Its product line is centered on organic teas and juice blends. Honest Teas recently launched a no calorie line that flavors its drinks with stevia.

Organic on the Cheap

20 Ways to Save Big Bucks on Organic Groceries

Quality costs more - it's not a theory, it's a fact. This applies to food as well. These days, everyone can benefit from saving money. Fortunately for you, there are numerous ways to significantly save money at the grocery register, and I've listed the top 20 resources. For added convenience, most of these resources are available within your own community (if you live in a city, you can also access many of these resources).

I care about all of my clients and I want to do everything in my power to ensure your success on your weight loss program. One of the easiest ways that I can do this is to help save you money so that you can lose weight and become healthier, without unloading your wallet.

1. Warehouse Shopping Clubs

Warehouse discount clubs have long been appreciated by the public for saving money on bulk items like paper towels and toilet tissue. Now you can add organic items to that list. Costco and BJ's are just two examples of warehouse stores that carry organic foods, such as meats, produce, dairy and eggs, soups and smoothies.

Chances are you probably already have a membership to one of these clubs. If you don't, you can get twice the value for half the price by splitting the membership with a friend or family member. Another option is to go shopping with someone who does. When you've finished shopping, give the person with the membership the money for your portion of the groceries!

If you live in a part of the country with a Super Walmart, be sure to check out their organic food and produce sections as well.

2. Farmer's Markets - Farmer Knows Best

Farmer's markets are a great resource within most

communities. The produce is local, the farmers are friendly, and the quality is outstanding. Many farmers don't us synthetic pesticides for their crops. Since crops are grown locally, they don't have to be transported far 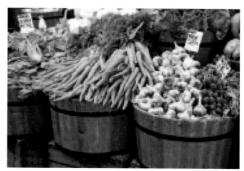 distances, which means that your food won't lose valuable nutrients during shipping. Best of all, if you have a question about a particular item, you can always ask the source directly!

Because produce is local, farmer's market prices are generally cheaper than organic and even conventional produce.

3. Community Supported Agriculture (CSA) - Produce Delivered to Your Door

CSAs are a new way to bring the farm to your door, literally. CSAs allow you to pay for a membership to purchase a share from a local farm for a season. Every week you'll receive a box of seasonal produce (the CSA will give you a list of the seasonal produce beforehand so you know how much of each item you'll be receiving). Prices for the membership (over the course of the season) are usually much lower than purchasing these items at a supermarket.

CSAs also offer other food items such as meats, dairy and homemade bread.

Not only is this option convenient, it's also cost effective. If you are a single person, you can save even more money by spitting the membership (and groceries) with another friend. To find a local CSA in your community, please visit: www.localharvest.org/csa

4. Go Directly to the Farm

Going directly to the farm allows you to purchase the freshest cuts of meats available - directly from the source. It's also the best place to get the cheapest price per pound. When supermarkets buy meats, they pay for shipping, packaging and the equipment to cool the meat. The store then passes these costs onto you, the consumer. Buying the meat directly from the farmer allows you to bypass the middle man, the grocery store, so that you can save money. This translates to less money per pound for your meat.

Many local farms feed their livestock grass and their chickens natural feed, so your food will still be nutritionally dense - for much less! If you want to confirm what the animals are eating, you can ask the farmer these questions directly.

Ask your family, friends and people in your neighborhood if they would like to split up the meat of a cow, pig, chicken, or lamb. Let them know that they will most likely pay   less per pound than going to the store - I'm sure you'll have no problem finding at least 10 willing participants. Many of these farms give you the option to buy dairy directly from them as well.

To find the closest farm to you, please visit: http://eatwild.com

5. Build Your Own Chicken Coop

As I've previously stated, pastured eggs are superior to conventional eggs in both nutrition and taste. If you live in the country you can make sure that you always have access to the freshest eggs around. How is this possible? By building your own chicken coop. You don't have to be an engineer to build a chicken coop; there are many do-it-yourself ebooks that can show you how to build your own chicken coop, step by step. For a great source visit: http://go.beyonddiet.com/chickencoop

6. Buy in Bulk Online

Buying meats in bulk is not something you only have to do at the farm; you can also buy bulk quality meats online. Buying online allows you to split the costs of the food with your friends and neighbors, and have the meat delivered directly to you. This is a great option if you're busy and don't have time to drive to your nearest farm.

7. Eat Fewer Processed Foods

This may seem like an obvious solution, but you'd be surprised at how much money you shell out on snacks and boxed foods. Cutting out processed foods is one of the easiest ways to save money on your grocery bill. You can test this option yourself. For one month, buy 1/2 to a 1/4 of the processed foods that you'd normally buy. At the end of the month, compare your previous month's bills with your bills for that month - I guarantee you'll see a difference.

8. Make More Delicious Meals at Home; Eat Out Less

Another easy way to save money is to make more of your meals at home. This includes lunches. On Sunday, set aside a few hours to cook your food for the week. Make about 6-8 simple meals, wrap them well and freeze them. Multiple meals allows you to rotate your meals, so you don't have to keep eating the same foods over and over again. Reward yourself by going out to dinner at your favorite restaurant at the end of the month, and bank the remainder of the money that you've saved.

9. Whole Nutrition = The Sum of All of The Parts

Use all of the parts of the animal, including the organs. Not only are these parts nutritionally dense, but they're cheap! Make sure that the organs are from pastured (grass fed) animals.

10. Is There a Butcher in the House?

Find a good quality butcher in your neighborhood for cheap bones and organs. Many people no longer make their own stocks, and many people do not eat organ meats (offal). Butchers will most likely throw these items away. They'll probably sell these items to you for very little money; if you're lucky, they may even give them to you for free! Remember to request grass fed bones and offal as they're the best choice.

11. Grow Your Own Veggies

One of the best ways to save money on produce is to grow your own at home. Growing your own garden is easier than you think; many people have been doing this as a hobby for years. Ebooks make tending your own garden easier than ever before.

I highly recommend "Food for Wealth" - If you are new to the world of organic gardening, this book breaks down the art of growing your own produce into simple steps. Once you've mastered the basics, I recommend a second book "Aquaponics4you." This book seriously improves your organic gardening techniques to yield more vegetables for your efforts. The combination will give you a one, two punch to getting the best value for your home grown organic garden.

Food4Wealth: www.food4wealth.com

Aquaponics4You: www.aquaponics4you.com

12. Co-ops

A food co-op is a collectively owned grocery store. A food co-op is a great central location for natural and organic foods more affordable for co-op members. Many co-op memberships require you to work at the store for a few hours a month in exchange for a free membership! Co-op members often receive discounts on many items within the store.

To find a natural co-op near you, please visit

http://www.coopdirectory.org

13. Private Label Brands

Look for sensibly priced Private Label Brands (PLB) at your supermarket. 365 Everyday is Whole Foods' PLB. The ingredients in most of their items are outstanding - in fact, all Whole Foods PLB items are natural, and most are organic! And the price can be a much as $3-4 less than their brand label counterpart!

14. Bone up on Marrow Bones

Marrow bones are inexpensive, luscious and super nutritious. They contain over 40% of monounsaturated fats (the same fats in olive oil and avocados). Many high class restaurants are now serving this treat as an expensive, decadent appetizer, but you can indulge for much less. Ask your local butcher, or the farmer if you are buying your meat directly from the farm to throw in some marrow bones with your order. Below is a recipe for roasted bone marrow:

Roasted Bone Marrow with Garlic

8-12 grass fed beef bones with marrow (3 to 4 pounds total)

1 cup fresh parsley, roughly chopped

1 head of garlic

2 shallots, thinly sliced

2 teaspoons capers

1 1/2 tablespoons extra virgin olive oil

2 teaspoons fresh lemon juice

Aztec Sea Salt

Sprouted Whole Grain bread, toasted

Preheat the oven to 375°F. Cut the top off the head of garlic and place in the middle of a sheet of aluminum foil. Drizzle with a couple teaspoons of olive oil and add a pinch of salt. Close the foil around the garlic, creating a tight pouch, and place the garlic into the oven for 45 minutes. Remove from the oven. Open the pouch and allow to cool for a couple of minutes. When the head of garlic is cool enough to the touch, squeeze out the warm, soft garlic and spread onto the toast with the marrow.

Preheat the oven to 450°F degrees. Place bones, cut side up, onto a foil-lined baking sheet or in an ovenproof cast iron skillet. Cook until the marrow is soft and has begun to separate from the bone - about 15 minutes. (Stop before the marrow begins to drizzle out). Meanwhile, combine parsley, shallots and capers into a small bowl. Just before the bones are ready, whisk together the olive oil and lemon juice and drizzle the dressing over the parsley mixture until the leaves are coated.

Place the roasted bones, parsley salad, salt and toast onto a large plate. To serve, scoop out the marrow, spread onto the toast, sprinkle with a tiny bit of salt and top with the parsley salad.

15. Dairy You Can Make at Home

If you are an avid cook or feel particularly adventurous in the kitchen, you can really stretch your dollars and make your own grass-fed yogurt and butter from pastured or raw milk.

For a DIY quality butter recipe, please refer to this link: http://www.foodrenegade.com/how-to-make-butter

Yogurt recipe provided by: http://nourishedkitchen.com/raw-milk-yogurt

16. Bake Your Own Bread

You can also make your own delicious, sprouted bread at home. For more money saving goodness, use this simple, yet hearty recipe.

Gluten Free Rice Bread Recipe

> 1 cup brown rice
>
> 7/8 cup water
>
> 1 egg
>
> 1 teaspoon baking powder
>
> 1/4 teaspoon

Soak the rice in the water
overnight (6-12 hours). Grind the rice and water mixture

in a blender until the rice particles in the batter reach the consistency of fine salt. Add egg, baking powder and salt to the batter, mix well.

Bake COVERED for 30 minutes in a well-oiled eight-inch iron skillet or a casserole dish (a well-seasoned cast iron skillet can't be beat for baking with rice).

17. Freeze It

Buy fruits and vegetables in bulk when they're in season. Double wrap the produce in freezer resistant wrapping, and place them in freezer bags to keep out freezer burn and lock in the flavor.

18. Bartering food with neighbors and friends

Save money on groceries by trading food items with your friends and neighbors in your community. This is also great if you have more food items than you or your family needs.

19. Online Coupons

You don't have to go searching your Sunday paper to clip coupons - unless you want to. There are great online resources like http://www.organicdeals.com/ and http://allnaturalsavings.com/, which provide many ways to save money on organic foods.

20. Have a Potluck Dinner!

This is the easiest and most social way to save money. Once a week (or however often you choose), have a healthy potluck dinner with your family, friends and neighbors using organic foods. Assign one or two dishes to each person. For the price of two side dishes, you'll have access to a full banquet of delicious, nutritious food!

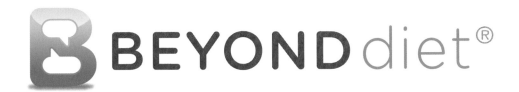

ADVANCED
MEAL PLANNING

Isabel De Los Rios

Getting Started

If you haven't yet watched the step-by-step video I've put together for you here, I strongly encourage you to take a few minutes to view it now. It's definitely the quickest and easiest way to start creating your own meal plans using Beyond Diet's Success Journal and Meal Tracker.

In the next section, I'm also going to give you a quick summary of the meal planning process, so you can refer back to it in the future...

Once you've completed Step 1 and Step 2 of the Beyond Diet program, you're ready to start planning your own meals in Step 3. And I'm going to make this super easy for you.

Meal Planning Tools

Take the Metabolism Test

Please take the Metabolism Test to determine your metabolism type - Protein Type, Carb Type, or Mixed Type. Next, read through the description of (and special considerations for) your metabolism type in the Metabolism Types chapter. You must understand why certain foods are ideal in order to make the best choices for your personal meal plan.

> 1. When I feel an
>
> **A.** heavy fatty foo
>
> **B.** fruit, vegetable

Use the Caloric Calculator

For proponents of metabolism typing, the only thing that matters is eating the ideal foods in the right proportions for your metabolism type - if you eat proteins, carbohydrates, and fats in certain ratios, then the number of calories is unimportant.

> Current Weight:
>
> 170
>
> Your Activity Level:
>
> ○ You exercise vigorousl
>
> ● You exercise moderat

But if a meal plan for weight loss isn't created with calorie counts, then on what is it based? Ideally, each of us would know when to eat and when to stop eating simply by "listening" to the body's hunger and satiation cues. Unfortunately though, most people who struggle with their weight have lost the ability to recognize when they are hungry or full and often eat when they feel stressed, bored, or pressured socially.

There is a way to account for this inability to listen to the body's cues, though. Estimate how many calories you need to consume daily using the Caloric Calculator. Even though the word calorie is loaded with bad (and wrong) connotations, this program suggests estimating your daily calorie requirements as a means to an end. Instead of actually counting calories though, this number is used to determine the correct number of servings of each food type for each meal.

Identify Your Ideal Food Ratios

Now it's time to identify your Ideal Food Ratios. On the Ideal Food Ratios chart, you see that different ratios of calories from proteins, carbohydrates, and fats are ideal for each metabolism type. Carb Types should have approximately 20% of their calories comes from proteins, 70% from carbohydrates, and 10% from fats. Mixed Types should have approximately 40% from proteins, 50% from carbohydrates, and 10% from fats; and Protein Types should eat approximately 45% of their calories from proteins, 35% from carbohydrates, and 20% from fats.

Your Metabolism Type:

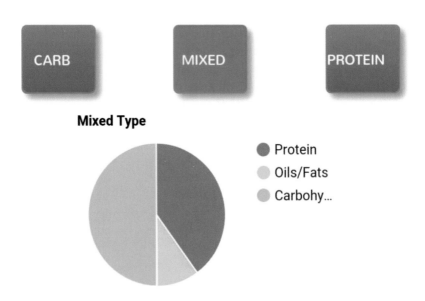

Mixed Type

- Protein
- Oils/Fats
- Carbohy...

For example, if you're a Mixed Type, each meal or snack (including your drink) should contain about half protein and half carbohydrates. (Note: The 10% fat would come from your protein source or from some added healthy oil.) Use the Allowable Servings Guide to create your own meal plans. You'll soon learn to tune in to your body's responses and learn when you have eaten the right amounts for you.

Determine Your Allowable Servings

Your Allowable Servings are determined using your daily calorie requirements and your metabolism type. Once you have completed these two steps, your servings will automatically be updated in your Success Journal.

Carb	**Mixed**	Protein

Meal	Lose Weight Goal (1600 calories / day)	Maintain Weight Goal (2000 calories / day)
Breakfast	2 Protein, 2 Carb	3 Protein, 2 Carb
Morning Snack	2 Protein, 2 Carb	2 Protein, 2 Carb

Identify Your Ideal Foods Using the Food Choices Chart

Eating the right kinds of food is just as important as eating the right quantities of food. Take a look at the Food Choices chart. Once you have taken the Metabolism Test, you will automatically see the chart for your metabolism type. The ideal foods for your type are shaded. Foods that are not highlighted in the charts should be avoided or eaten only occasionally. For example, an orange - generally thought of as a healthy food - will help balance a Carb Type but may push a Protein Type out of balance.

Because each person is unique, these charts must be considered as a starting point to find which foods are best for you. For example, I always test as a Protein Type but feel pretty good eating cucumbers - one food that most Protein Types typically should avoid. When I feel lethargic soon after eating or hungry an hour later, I know I've eaten a food that isn't good for me (or that my meal didn't have the correct protein-to-carbohydrate ratio). Again, these charts are only starting points to determine which foods might be best for you. Pay attention to how you feel after eating; track symptoms that might be related to the foods you eat in your Success Journal.

Carb   **Fat**   Protein

⌄ Fat

Servings	Food
1.00 tsp	olive oil
1.00 tsp	fish oil
1.00 tsp	cod liver oil
1.00 tsp	flax seed oil
1.00 tsp	raw butter
1.00 oz	avocado
Free	coconut oil
1.00 oz	raw cheese
1.00 tsp	avocado oil
1.00 tsp	ghee

Planning Your Meals

Now it's time to put all the pieces together to create a truly personal meal plan - one that meets the needs of your metabolism type and includes foods that you enjoy. Let's start with an example. If you are a Protein Type and, according to the Allowable Servings Guide, you require three protein servings at Breakfast, here are some possible options from the Protein chart:

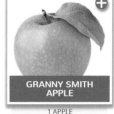

- 2 eggs and 1 slice of bacon

- 3 ounces of meat or poultry (possibly leftovers from the night before)

- Or something else from the chart

A Protein Type may also require one carbohydrate serving at Breakfast. Possible options from the Carbohydrate chart include:

- 1 medium apple

- 1 cup of spinach (e.g., in an omelet)

- 1 cup of cooked oatmeal

- Or something else from the chart

For a Snack, a Protein Type may require three protein servings and one carbohydrate serving, which could be:

- 1 1/2 ounces of raw almonds and 1 medium apple

- 3 ounces of leftover turkey and 1/2 cup each of celery and carrots

- Or something else from the chart

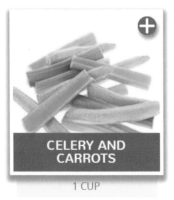

CELERY AND CARROTS

1 CUP

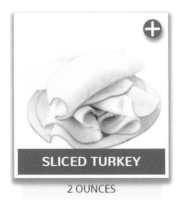

SLICED TURKEY

2 OUNCES

The process of creating meals for Lunch and Dinner is the same as for Breakfast and Snacks, but you will add Fat servings, as indicated on the Allowable Servings Guide. Don't give in to society's urging to avoid all fats, thinking that doing so will help you lose weight faster. In fact, you must consume a substantial amount of healthy fat each day to lose weight, keep energy levels high, and feel satiated. (The Chapter on Fats addresses this topic in detail.) Also, the Recipe Guide and Recipes section will help you cook up some healthy and delicious meals.

Remember, the information listed in the Allowable Servings Guide and Food Choices chart are only suggestions and starting points. If you feel hungry at any time, you will need to adjust your meal plan in some way. Depending on your metabolism type, you might add a bit more protein, carbohydrate, or fat to a meal (to adjust the protein-carbohydrate-fat ratio slightly) or add another Snack to your day (amking sure to keep that meal balanced and appropriate for your type) until you feel satiated and energized. And if something you eat makes you feel lethargic, avoid it.

Adding Food and Recipes to Your Meal Tracker

From the Beyond Diet Member Home Page, click "Success Journal" in the drop down menu in upper right hand corner, or click the blue tile labeled "My Success Journal."

Once you're inside your Success Journal, click the orange tile labeled "Meals" to get started.

MY SUCCESS JOURNAL

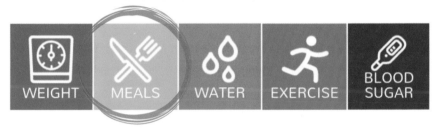

WEIGHT   MEALS   WATER   EXERCISE   BLOOD SUGAR

Your Meal Tracker defaults to today's date, but you can change the date you want to plan meals for by clicking "Select Another Date" at the top of the page.

Friday, June 17

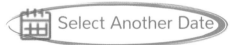 Select Another Date

⊕ Add   **Breakfast**   P F C

Breakfast Total   0/2 0/0 0/2

(actual/goal)

Since you've already completed the Metabolism Test, your recommended allowable servings for each meal and snack will be pre-populated below the Protein (P), Fat (F), and Carb (C) headers.

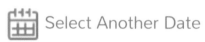

Friday, June 17

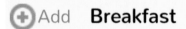 Select Another Date

⊕ Add **Breakfast**   P F C

Breakfast Total   0/2 0/0 0/2

(actual/goal)

Now you're ready to start planning your meals!

You have three different options for adding foods and recipes to your Meal Tracker. You can…

- add an individual BD-approved food,

- add an entire recipe from the Recipe section,

- or add an individual unapproved food.

Start by clicking "+Add" to the meal you want to plan first: Breakfast, Morning Snack, Lunch, Afternoon Snack, or Dinner.

 Breakfast

Breakfast Total   0/2 0/0 0/2

(actual/goal)

When you click "+Add" you will be directed to a new page where you can add a specific food and quantity, or a full recipe.

Decide whether you want to add a Beyond Diet food, Beyond Diet recipe, or an unapproved food to your Meal Tracker and scroll down to the appropriate field. Type in the name of the individual food or recipe you want to add.

- BD FOOD: Enter the name of the food and select it from the drop down window. Next, enter the quantity. The servings of Protein, Fat, and Carb for that food will be automatically updated.

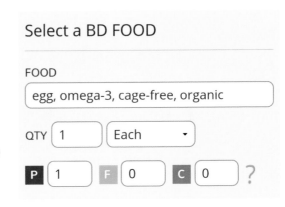

- RECIPE: Enter the name of the recipe and select it from the drop down window. Next, enter the number of servings. The servings of Protein, Fat, and Carb for that food will be automatically updated.

- UNAPPROVED FOOD: Enter the name of the food and the quantity. Protein, Fat, and Carb servings are NOT automatically calculated for unapproved foods, so go ahead and fill these fields in to the best of your ability using the information in the video below.

Enter an UNAPPROVED FOOD

FOOD

French fries

QUANTITY | 1 cup

Not Automatically Calculated

P [ ] F [ ] C [ ] ?

ADD FOOD TO BREAKFAST

Now, click the blue button labeled "ADD FOOD/RECIPE TO MEAL" and you will be returned to your Meal Tracker, and be able to see the food or recipe you just added.

Continue adding the individual foods or recipes you plan to eat until your allowable servings for Proteins, Fats, and Carbs are met for that meal.

That's it!

Meal Planning Next Steps

You've just received a bunch of super-important information on the meal planning process.

As you transition to Step 3 of Beyond Diet, you may be feeling a wide range of emotions - anything from excitement to hesitation to relief, or even nervousness - about adjusting to your healthy new lifestyle, and everything that goes along with it.

But, no matter how you're feeling at the moment, stick with me, because right now I'm going to help you overcome any lingering doubts or concerns you may have at this point.

I have to tell you, the first time I sat down to create a healthy meal plan, I was completely overwhelmed. (I actually think I had a minor panic attack for a minute.) I didn't even know where to begin!

Luckily for you, you have an experienced, certified nutritionist by your side to show you the exact steps you need to be successful.

Using the tools provided in this guide - and a little patience and practice - you will get the hang of it, I promise!

Want to See How to Plan Meals in Half the Time?

Visit http://go.beyonddiet.com/Step3BDM

Metabolism Type Test

Adapted from The Metabolic Typing Diet (Wolcott and Fahey 2000, 135), this simple test is the most basic way to determine your metabolism type.

Circle the answer that best completes the following 25 statements according to how you actually feel, not how you think you should feel. If you don't usually pay attention to your body's cues before and after eating, then do so for a few days (while continuing your present eating habits) before taking the test. To ensure a valid result, be honest and do not skip any questions!

Instructions for scoring follow.

Questions

1. When I feel anxious, angry, or irritable,

   A. heavy fatty foods such as meat or salty nuts make me feel better.

   B. fruit, vegetables, or fruit juice makes me feel better.

2. I feel best when I eat the following for breakfast:

   A. sausage, eggs, and/or bacon.

   B. cereal, fruit, and/or toast.

3. If I attended a buffet and could eat whatever I wanted (all health rules aside), I would choose

   A. steak, pork chops, ribs, gravy, and a salad with creamy dressing.

   B. chicken, turkey, fish, vegetables, and a dessert.

4. I feel best when the temperature is

   A. cool or cold; I don't like hot weather.

   B. warm or hot; I don't like cold weather.

5. Coffee makes me feel

   A. jittery, jumpy, nervous, hyper, shaky, or hungry.

   B. okay, as long as I don't drink too much.

6. In the morning, I am

   A. hungry and ready to eat breakfast.

   B. not hungry and don't feel like eating.

7. At midday, I am

   A. hungry and ready to eat lunch.

   B. not noticeably hungry and have to be reminded to eat.

8. In the evening, I am

   A. hungry and ready to eat dinner.

   B. not noticeably hungry and have to be reminded to eat.

9. I concentrate best if I have eaten a meal that includes

   A. meat and fatty foods.

   B. fruits, vegetables, and grains.

10. When I have cravings, I tend to want

   A. salty and fatty snacks (peanuts, cheese, or potato chips).

   B. baked goods or other carbs (bread, cereal, or crackers).

11. When I eat sugar or a sugary snack,

   A. I feel a rush of energy, then am likely to crash and feel fatigued.

   B. my energy levels are restored.

12. If dessert is served,

   A. I can take it or leave it; I would rather have cheese, chips, or popcorn.

   B. I definitely will indulge; I like to have something sweet after a meal.

13. If I have a dessert, I most often choose

   A. cheesecake or creamy French pastries.

   B. cakes, cookies, or candies.

14. For dinner, I feel best (satiated) after eating

   A. steak and vegetables.

   B. skinless chicken breast, rice, and a salad.

15. I sleep best if my dinner is

   A. heavy and includes more proteins.

   B. light and includes more carbohydrates.

16. I wake up feeling well rested if

   A. I don't eat sweets in the evening.

   B. I eat sweets in the evening.

17. I feel best during the day if I eat

   A. small meals frequently, or three meals a day plus some snacks.

   B. two to three meals a day and no snacks; I can last pretty long without eating.

18. I describe myself as someone who

   A. loves to eat; food is a central part of my life.

   B. is not very concerned with food; I may forget to eat at times.

19. If I skip a meal, I feel

    A. irritable, jittery, weak, tired, or depressed.

    B. okay; it doesn't really bother me.

20. If I had fruit and low-fat cottage cheese for lunch, I would feel

    A. hungry, irritable, and sleepy soon after.

    B. satisfied and probably could go until dinner after that.

21. During the day, I feel hungry

    A. often and need to eat several times a day.

    B. rarely and have a weak appetite.

22. I would describe myself as someone who is more

    A. extroverted—I am a very social person.

    B. introverted—I usually keep to myself.

23. When a food or meal is very salty,

    A. I love it!

    B. I don't enjoy it.

24. If I get hungry midafternoon, I feel best (more energized) after eating

    A. cheese and nuts.

    B. something sweet.

25. After exercising, I feel best if I eat

A. a protein shake or food that contains protein.

B. a high-sugar drink or food, such as a Gatorade or a banana.

Scoring

First, count how many times you circled A and B to determine your scores:

Total number of A answers = _____

Total number of B answers = _____

Next, referring to these scores, select your metabolism type classification according to the following criteria:

- If your A score is 5 or more points higher than your B score (e.g., A = 15, B = 10), then you are a **Protein Type**.

- If your B score is 5 or more points higher than your A score (e.g., A = 10, B = 15), then you are a **Carb Type**.

- If your A and B scores are within 3 points of each other (e.g., A = 14, B = 11), then you are a **Mixed Type**.

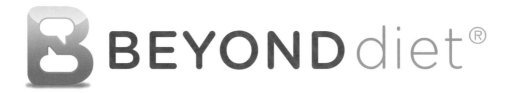

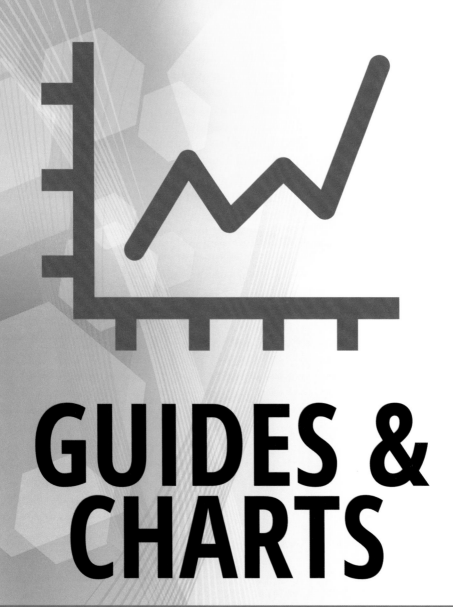

GUIDES & CHARTS

Isabel De Los Rios

Cooking with Fats

The following guide to commonly used culinary fats will help you choose the proper fats for each type of cooking according to their smoke points (Chek 2004, 73). Always use unrefined organic oils and raw organic butter!

No-heat fats should never be used for cooking:

- borage oil
- fish oil or cod liver oil
- flax seed oil
- hemp seed oil

Low-heat fats should be heated to no more than 212°F:

- pumpkin oil
- safflower oil
- sunflower oil

Medium-heat fats should be heated to no more than 325°F (light sautéing):

- hazelnut oil
- olive oil
- pistachio oil
- sesame oil

High-heat fats should be heated to no more than 375°F (frying or browning):

- butter (for cooking at medium-high heat only; do not allow to turn brown)

- coconut oil

- ghee or clarified butter

Allowable Servings Guide

Type	Mixed	Carb	Protein
Meal	1,400 calories/day		
Breakfast	2 Protein 2 Carb	1 Protein 2 Carb	3 Protein 1 Carb
Snack	2 Protein 2 Carb	1 Protein 2 Carb	2 Protein 1 Carb
Lunch	3 Protein 1 Carb 1 Fat	3 Protein 2 Carb 1 Fat	3 Protein 1 Carb 2 Fat
Snack	2 Protein 1 Carb	2 Protein 2 Carb	2 Protein 1 Carb
Dinner	3 Protein 2 Carb 2 Fat	3 Protein 2 Carb 1 Fat	4 Protein 1 Carb 2 Fat
	1,600 calories/day		
Breakfast	2 Protein 2 Carb	1 Protein 2 Carb	3 Protein 1 Carb
Snack	2 Protein 2 Carb	1 Protein 2 Carb	2 Protein 1 Carb
Lunch	4 Protein 1 Carb 1 Fat	4 Protein 2 Carb 1 Fat	4 Protein 1 Carb 2 Fat
Snack	2 Protein 1 Carb	2 Protein 2 Carb	2 Protein 1 Carb
Dinner	4 Protein 2 Carb 2 Fat	4 Protein 2 Carb 1 Fat	5 Protein 1 Carb 2 Fat

Note: **Refer to the Food Choice charts to choose the appropriate foods in each category for your metabolism type.**

Type	Mixed	Carb	Protein
Meal	1,800 calories/day		
Breakfast	2 Protein 2 Carb	1 Protein 2 Carb	3 Protein 1 Carb
Snack	2 Protein 2 Carb	2 Protein 2 Carb	3 Protein 1 Carb
Lunch	4 Protein 2 Carb 1 Fat	4 Protein 2 Carb 1 Fat	4 Protein 1 Carb 2 Fat
Snack	2 Protein 1 Carb	2 Protein 3 Carb	2 Protein 1 Carb
Dinner	5 Protein 2 Carb 2 Fat	4 Protein 2 Carb 1 Fat	5 Protein 1 Carb 2 Fat
	2,000 calories/day		
Breakfast	3 Protein 2 Carb	2 Protein 3 Carb	3 Protein 1 Carb
Snack	2 Protein 2 Carb	2 Protein 2 Carb	3 Protein 1 Carb
Lunch	4 Protein 2 Carb 1 Fat	4 Protein 2 Carb 1 Fat	5 Protein 1 Carb 2 Fat
Snack	2 Protein 1 Carb	2 Protein 3 Carb	3 Protein 1 Carb
Dinner	5 Protein 2 Carb 2 Fat	4 Protein 2 Carb 1 Fat	5 Protein 1 Carb 2 Fat

Note: **Refer to the Food Choice charts to choose the appropriate foods in each category for your metabolism type.**

Type	Mixed	Carb	Protein
Meal	2,200 calories/day		
Breakfast	3 Protein 2 Carb	2 Protein 3 Carb	4 Protein 1 Carb
Snack	3 Protein 2 Carb	2 Protein 3 Carb	3 Protein 1 Carb
Lunch	4 Protein 2 Carb 1 Fat	4 Protein 3 Carb 1 Fat	5 Protein 1 Carb 2 Fat
Snack	2 Protein 2 Carb	2 Protein 3 Carb	4 Protein 1 Carb
Dinner	5 Protein 2 Carb 2 Fat	4 Protein 2 Carb 1 Fat	5 Protein 1 Carb 2 Fat
	2,400 calories/day		
Breakfast	3 Protein 2 Carb	2 Protein 3 Carb	4 Protein 2 Carb
Snack	3 Protein 2 Carb	2 Protein 3 Carb	3 Protein 1 Carb
Lunch	4 Protein 3 Carb 2 Fat	4 Protein 3 Carb 2 Fat	5 Protein 1 Carb 2 Fat
Snack	3 Protein 2 Carb	2 Protein 3 Carb	4 Protein 1 Carb
Dinner	5 Protein 2 Carb 2 Fat	4 Protein 3 Carb 1 Fat	6 Protein 1 Carb 2 Fat

Note: **Refer to the Food Choice charts to choose the appropriate foods in each category for your metabolism type.**

Food Choices

For all charts in this section, the "best bet" food items are shaded in blue.

Carb Types: Protein Choices

Serving	Meats	Serving	Seafood (cont'd)	Serving	Dairy and Eggs
1 slice	bacon (pork)	1 oz (28 g)	cod	1	egg
1 slice	bacon (beef)	1 oz (28 g)	crabmeat	¼ cup (60 g)	cottage cheese
1 oz (28 g)	beef	1 oz (28 g)	crayfish	2 oz (56 g)	Greek yogurt
1 oz (28 g)	buffalo	1 oz (28 g)	flounder		**Nuts[1] and Seeds**
1 oz (28 g)	lamb	1 oz (28 g)	grouper	½ oz (14 g)	almonds
1 oz (28 g)	liver (beef or chicken)	1 oz (28 g)	halibut	½ oz (14 g)	Brazil nuts
1 oz (28 g)	pork (lean)	1 oz (28 g)	herring	½ oz (14 g)	cashews
1 oz (28 g)	rabbit	1 oz (28 g)	lobster meat	½ oz (14 g)	chestnuts
1 oz (28 g)	venison	1 oz (28 g)	mackerel	½ oz (14 g)	filberts
	Poultry	1 oz (28 g)	mahi mahi	½ oz (14 g)	hickory nuts
1 slice	bacon (turkey)	1 oz (28 g)	mussels	½ oz (14 g)	macadamia nuts
1 oz (28 g)	chicken (dark)	1 oz (28 g)	octopus	½ oz (14 g)	peanuts[2]
1 oz (28 g)	chicken (white)	1 oz (28 g)	perch (freshwater)	½ oz (14 g)	pecans
1 oz (28 g)	duck	1 oz (28 g)	rockfish	½ oz (14 g)	pine nuts
1 oz (28 g)	goose	1 oz (28 g)	roughy	½ oz (14 g)	pistachios
1 oz (28 g)	Cornish hen	1 oz (28 g)	salmon	½ oz (14 g)	pumpkin seeds
1 oz (28 g)	pheasant	1 oz (28 g)	sardines	½ oz (14 g)	sunflower seeds
1 oz (28 g)	quail	1 oz (28 g)	shrimp	½ oz (14 g)	walnuts
1 oz (28 g)	sausage (chicken)	1 oz (28 g)	snapper	1 Tbsp (15 mL)	nut butter[3]
1 oz (28 g)	turkey (dark)	1 oz (28 g)	squid		
1 oz (28 g)	turkey (white)	1 oz (28 g)	swordfish		
	Seafood	1 oz (28 g)	trout		
1 oz (28 g)	abalone	1 oz (28 g)	tuna (white)		
1 oz (28 g)	anchovy	1 oz (28 g)	whitefish		
1 oz (28 g)	bass (freshwater)				
1 oz (28 g)	bass (sea)				
1 oz (28 g)	catfish				
1 oz (28 g)	caviar				
1 oz (28 g)	clams				

[1] All nuts and seeds must be raw.

[2] Peanuts are legumes but are listed with tree nuts here for ease of presentation.

[3] Varieties of nut butter include almond, cashew, macadamia nut, and walnut.

Carb Types: Carbohydrate Choices

Serving	Bread	Serving	Fruits (cont'd)	Serving	Dairy and Eggs
1 slice	SWG** bread	1 cup (150 g)	casaba melon[1]	2 cups (300 g)	rhubarb
½	SWG** roll	17	cherries	1 cup (150 g)	strawberries
½	SWG** English muffin	1 cup (150 g)	cranberries	2	tangerines (small)
1	SWG** wrap (small)	1 cup (150 g)	currants	1	tomato (large)
1 slice	rice bread	1	date	1 cup (150 g)	watermelon
1 slice	spelt bread	¾ cup (111g)	elderberries		
10	rice crackers	2	figs (large)		
2	rye crackers	1 cup (150 g)	gooseberries		
	Grains*	1	grapefruit (small)		
½ cup (75g)	brown or wild rice	17-20	grapes		
½ cup (75g)	amaranth	1 cup (150 g)	guava		
½ cup (75g)	barley	1 cup (150 g)	honeydew melon		
½ cup (75g)	buckwheat	2	kiwifruit (medium)		
½ cup (75g)	non-GMO corn	6	kumquat[2]		
½ cup (75g)	kamut	free	lemons		
½ cup (75g)	millet	free	limes		
1 cup (150g)	oatmeal	1 cup (150 g)	loganberries[3]		
½ cup (75g)	quinoa	½	mango		
½ cup (75g)	rye	2	nectarines		
½ cup (75g)	spelt	1	orange (large)		
½ cup (75g)	SWG** cereal	½	papaya (large)		
½ cup (75g)	raw granola	1	peach (medium)		
	Fruits*	1	pear (medium)		
1	apple (medium)	2	persimmons		
4	apricots (small)	1 cup (150 g)	pineapple		
½	banana	2	plums (small)		
1 cup (150 g)	blackberries	1	pomegranate (sm)		
1 cup (150 g)	blueberries	4	prunes (small)		
1 cup (150 g)	boysenberries	2 Tbsp (30 g)	raisins		
1 cup (150 g)	cantaloupe	1 cup (150 g)	raspberries		

* Serving sizes of grains and legumes are measured cooked, those of fruits and vegetables are measured raw

** SWG = Sprouted Whole Grain (e.g. Ezekiel 4:9 products)

Free = Use as needed for seasoning

[1] Similar to a cantaloupe

[2] similar to an orange but small like a grape

[3] cross between a blackberry and raspberry

Carb Types: Carbohydrate Choices

Serving	Legumes*	Serving	Low-Starch Veg*	Serving	Dairy and Eggs
½ cup (75g)	adzuki beans	1	artichoke	1 cup (150 g)	salad greens[2]
½ cup (75g)	black beans	1 cup (150 g)	asparagus	1 cup (30 g)	spinach
½ cup (75g)	black-eyed beans	½ cup (75g)	bamboo shoots	½ cup (75g)	squash (winter)[4]
½ cup (75g)	fava beans	1 cup (150 g)	bok choy	½ cup (75g)	turnip
½ cup (75g)	garbanzo beans	1 cup (150 g)	broccoli	1 cup (150 g)	zucchini
½ cup (75g)	great Northern beans	1 cup (150 g)	Brussels sprouts		
½ cup (75g)	green beans	1 cup (150 g)	cabbage		
½ cup (75g)	green peas	1 cup (150 g)	cauliflower		
½ cup (75g)	lentils	1 cup (150 g)	celery		
½ cup (75g)	lima beans	1 cup (150 g)	cucumber		
½ cup (75g)	mung beans	1 cup (150 g)	daikon[1]		
½ cup (75g)	navy beans	1 cup (150 g)	eggplant		
½ cup (75g)	pink beans	1 cup (150 g)	fennel		
½ cup (75g)	pinto beans	free	garlic		
½ cup (75g)	red beans	free	ginger root		
½ cup (75g)	white beans	1 cup (150 g)	jicama		
	Dairy	1 cup (150 g)	kale		
½ cup (75g)	milk (raw)	free	lettuce[2]		
6 oz (168 g)	plain yogurt	1 cup (150 g)	mushrooms		
	High-Starch Veg*	1 cup (150 g)	okra		
1 cup (150 g)	beets	5	olives		
1 cup (150 g)	carrots	1	onion (medium)		
½ cup (75g)	Jerusalem artichoke	1 cup (150 g)	pepper (bell)		
½ cup (75g)	parsnips	free	pepper (hot)		
½ cup (75g)	potato (white)	½ cup (75g)	pumpkin		
½ cup (75g)	potato (sweet)	½ cup (75g)	radishes		
¼ cup (60g)	water chestnuts	½ cup (75g)	rutabaga[3]		

* Serving sizes of grains and legumes are measured cooked, those of fruits and vegetables are measured raw

Free = Use as needed for seasoning

[1] Japanese radish

[2] Any but iceberg

[3] Similar to a turnip

[4] Orange-fleshed squashes (e.g. acorn, butternut, and kabocha)

Protein Types: Protein Choices

Serving	Meats	Serving	Seafood (cont'd)	Serving	Dairy and Eggs
1 slice	bacon (pork)	1 oz (28 g)	cod	1	egg
1 slice	bacon (beef)	1 oz (28 g)	crabmeat	¼ cup (60 g)	cottage cheese
1 oz (28 g)	beef	1 oz (28 g)	crayfish	2 oz (56 g)	Greek yogurt
1 oz (28 g)	buffalo	1 oz (28 g)	grouper		Nuts[1] and Seeds
1 oz (28 g)	lamb	1 oz (28 g)	halibut	½ oz (14 g)	almonds
1 oz (28 g)	liver (beef or chicken)	1 oz (28 g)	herring	½ oz (14 g)	Brazil nuts
1 oz (28 g)	pork (lean)	1 oz (28 g)	lobster meat	½ oz (14 g)	cashews
1 oz (28 g)	rabbit	1 oz (28 g)	mackerel	½ oz (14 g)	chestnuts
1 oz (28 g)	venison	1 oz (28 g)	mahi mahi	½ oz (14 g)	filberts
	Poultry	1 oz (28 g)	mussels	½ oz (14 g)	hickory nuts
1 slice	bacon (turkey)	1 oz (28 g)	octopus	½ oz (14 g)	macadamia nuts
1 oz (28 g)	chicken (dark)	1 oz (28 g)	perch (ocean)	½ oz (14 g)	peanuts[2]
1 oz (28 g)	chicken (white)	1 oz (28 g)	pompano	½ oz (14 g)	pecans
1 oz (28 g)	duck	1 oz (28 g)	rockfish	½ oz (14 g)	pine nuts
1 oz (28 g)	goose	1 oz (28 g)	roughy	½ oz (14 g)	pistachios
1 oz (28 g)	Cornish hen	1 oz (28 g)	salmon	½ oz (14 g)	pumpkin seeds
1 oz (28 g)	pheasant	1 oz (28 g)	sardines	½ oz (14 g)	sunflower seeds
1 oz (28 g)	quail	1 oz (28 g)	scallops	½ oz (14 g)	walnuts
1 oz (28 g)	sausage (chicken)	1 oz (28 g)	shark	1 Tbsp (15 mL)	nut butter[3]
1 oz (28 g)	turkey (dark)	1 oz (28 g)	shrimp		
1 oz (28 g)	turkey (white)	1 oz (28 g)	snapper	[1] All nuts and seeds must be raw.	
	Seafood	1 oz (28 g)	squid		
1 oz (28 g)	abalone	1 oz (28 g)	swordfish	[2] Peanuts are legumes but are listed with tree nuts here for ease of presentation.	
1 oz (28 g)	anchovy	1 oz (28 g)	trout		
1 oz (28 g)	bass (freshwater)	1 oz (28 g)	tuna (dark)		
1 oz (28 g)	bass (sea)	1 oz (28 g)	whitefish	[3] Varieties of nut butter include almond, cashew, macadamia nut, and walnut.	
1 oz (28 g)	catfish				
1 oz (28 g)	caviar				
1 oz (28 g)	clams				

Protein Types: Carbohydrate Choices

Serving	Bread	Serving	Fruits (cont'd)	Serving	Dairy and Eggs
1 slice	SWG** bread	1 cup (150 g)	casaba melon[1]	2 cups (300 g)	rhubarb
½	SWG** roll	17	cherries	1 cup (150 g)	strawberries
½	SWG** English muffin	1 cup (150 g)	cranberries	2	tangerines (small)
1	SWG** wrap (small)	1 cup (150 g)	currants	1	tomato (large)
1 slice	rice bread	1	date	1 cup (150 g)	watermelon
1 slice	spelt bread	¾ cup (111g)	elderberries		
10	rice crackers	2	figs (large)		
2	rye crackers	1 cup (150 g)	gooseberries		
	Grains*	1	grapefruit (small)		
½ cup (75g)	brown or wild rice	17-20	grapes		
½ cup (75g)	amaranth	1 cup (150 g)	guava		
½ cup (75g)	barley	1 cup (150 g)	honeydew melon		
½ cup (75g)	buckwheat	2	kiwifruit (medium)		
½ cup (75g)	non-GMO corn	6	kumquat[2]		
½ cup (75g)	kamut	free	lemons		
½ cup (75g)	millet	free	limes		
1 cup (150g)	oatmeal	1 cup (150 g)	loganberries[3]		
½ cup (75g)	quinoa	½	mango		
½ cup (75g)	rye	2	nectarines		
½ cup (75g)	spelt	1	orange (large)		
½ cup (75g)	SWG** cereal	½	papaya (large)		
½ cup (75g)	raw granola	1	peach (medium)		
	Fruits*	1	pear (medium)		
1	apple (medium)	2	persimmons		
4	apricots (small)	1 cup (150 g)	pineapple		
2 oz (56 g)	avocado	2	plums (small)		
½	banana	1	pomegranate (sm)		
1 cup (150 g)	blackberries	4	prunes (small)		
1 cup (150 g)	blueberries	2 Tbsp (30 g)	raisins		
1 cup (150 g)	boysenberries	1 cup (150 g)	raspberries		
1 cup (150 g)	cantaloupe				

* Serving sizes of grains and legumes are measured cooked, those of fruits and vegetables are measured raw

** SWG = Sprouted Whole Grain (e.g. Ezekiel 4:9 products)

Free = Use as needed for seasoning

[1] Similar to a cantaloupe

[2] similar to an orange but small like a grape

[3] cross between a blackberry and raspberry

Protein Types: Carbohydrate Choices

Serving	Legumes*	Serving	Low-Starch Veg*	Serving	Dairy and Eggs
½ cup (75g)	adzuki beans	1	artichoke	1 cup (150 g)	salad greens[2]
½ cup (75g)	black beans	1 cup (150 g)	asparagus	1 cup (30 g)	spinach
½ cup (75g)	black-eyed beans	½ cup (75g)	bamboo shoots	½ cup (75g)	squash (winter)[4]
½ cup (75g)	fava beans	1 cup (150 g)	bok choy	½ cup (75g)	turnip
½ cup (75g)	garbanzo beans	1 cup (150 g)	broccoli	1 cup (150 g)	zucchini
½ cup (75g)	great Northern beans	1 cup (150 g)	Brussels sprouts		
½ cup (75g)	green beans	1 cup (150 g)	cabbage		
½ cup (75g)	green peas	1 cup (150 g)	cauliflower		
½ cup (75g)	lentils	1 cup (150 g)	celery		
½ cup (75g)	lima beans	1 cup (150 g)	cucumber		
½ cup (75g)	mung beans	1 cup (150 g)	daikon[1]		
½ cup (75g)	navy beans	1 cup (150 g)	eggplant		
½ cup (75g)	pink beans	1 cup (150 g)	fennel		
½ cup (75g)	pinto beans	free	garlic		
½ cup (75g)	red beans	free	ginger root		
½ cup (75g)	white beans	1 cup (150 g)	jicama		
	Dairy	1 cup (150 g)	kale		
½ cup (75g)	milk (raw)	free	lettuce[2]		
6 oz (168 g)	plain yogurt	1 cup (150 g)	mushrooms		
	High-Starch Veg*	1 cup (150 g)	okra		
1 cup (150 g)	beets	5	olives		
1 cup (150 g)	carrots	1	onion (medium)		
½ cup (75g)	Jerusalem artichoke	1 cup (150 g)	pepper (bell)		
½ cup (75g)	parsnips	free	pepper (hot)		
½ cup (75g)	potato (white)	½ cup (75g)	pumpkin		
½ cup (75g)	potato (sweet)	½ cup (75g)	radishes		
¼ cup (60g)	water chestnuts	½ cup (75g)	rutabaga[3]		

* Serving sizes of grains and legumes are measured cooked, those of fruits and vegetables are measured raw

Free = Use as needed for seasoning

[1] Japanese radish

[2] Any but iceberg

[3] Similar to a turnip

[4] Orange-fleshed squashes (e.g. acorn, butternut, and kabocha)

Mixed Types: Protein Choices

Serving	Meats	Serving	Seafood (cont'd)	Serving	Dairy and Eggs
1 slice	bacon (pork)	1 oz (28 g)	cod	1	egg
1 slice	bacon (beef)	1 oz (28 g)	crabmeat	¼ cup (60 g)	cottage cheese
1 oz (28 g)	beef	1 oz (28 g)	crayfish	2 oz (56 g)	Greek yogurt
1 oz (28 g)	buffalo	1 oz (28 g)	grouper		**Nuts[1] and Seeds**
1 oz (28 g)	lamb	1 oz (28 g)	halibut	½ oz (14 g)	almonds
1 oz (28 g)	liver (beef or chicken)	1 oz (28 g)	herring	½ oz (14 g)	Brazil nuts
1 oz (28 g)	pork (lean)	1 oz (28 g)	lobster meat	½ oz (14 g)	cashews
1 oz (28 g)	rabbit	1 oz (28 g)	mackerel	½ oz (14 g)	chestnuts
1 oz (28 g)	venison	1 oz (28 g)	mahi mahi	½ oz (14 g)	filberts
	Poultry	1 oz (28 g)	mussels	½ oz (14 g)	hickory nuts
1 slice	bacon (turkey)	1 oz (28 g)	octopus	½ oz (14 g)	macadamia nuts
1 oz (28 g)	chicken (dark)	1 oz (28 g)	perch (ocean)	½ oz (14 g)	peanuts[2]
1 oz (28 g)	chicken (white)	1 oz (28 g)	pompano	½ oz (14 g)	pecans
1 oz (28 g)	duck	1 oz (28 g)	rockfish	½ oz (14 g)	pine nuts
1 oz (28 g)	goose	1 oz (28 g)	roughy	½ oz (14 g)	pistachios
1 oz (28 g)	Cornish hen	1 oz (28 g)	salmon	½ oz (14 g)	pumpkin seeds
1 oz (28 g)	pheasant	1 oz (28 g)	sardines	½ oz (14 g)	sunflower seeds
1 oz (28 g)	quail	1 oz (28 g)	scallops	½ oz (14 g)	walnuts
1 oz (28 g)	sausage (chicken)	1 oz (28 g)	shark	1 Tbsp (15 mL)	nut butter[3]
1 oz (28 g)	turkey (dark)	1 oz (28 g)	shrimp		
1 oz (28 g)	turkey (white)	1 oz (28 g)	snapper		
	Seafood	1 oz (28 g)	squid		
1 oz (28 g)	abalone	1 oz (28 g)	swordfish		
1 oz (28 g)	anchovy	1 oz (28 g)	trout		
1 oz (28 g)	bass (freshwater)	1 oz (28 g)	tuna (dark)		
1 oz (28 g)	bass (sea)	1 oz (28 g)	whitefish		
1 oz (28 g)	catfish				
1 oz (28 g)	caviar				
1 oz (28 g)	clams				

[1] All nuts and seeds must be raw.

[2] Peanuts are legumes but are listed with tree nuts here for ease of presentation.

[3] Varieties of nut butter include almond, cashew, macadamia nut, and walnut.

Mixed Types: Carbohydrate Choices

Serving	Bread	Serving	Fruits (cont'd)	Serving	Dairy and Eggs
1 slice	SWG** bread	1 cup (150 g)	casaba melon[1]	2 cups (300 g)	rhubarb
½	SWG** roll	17	cherries	1 cup (150 g)	strawberries
½	SWG** English muffin	1 cup (150 g)	cranberries	2	tangerines (small)
1	SWG** wrap (small)	1 cup (150 g)	currants	1	tomato (large)
1 slice	rice bread	1	date	1 cup (150 g)	watermelon
1 slice	spelt bread	¾ cup (111g)	elderberries		
10	rice crackers	2	figs (large)		
2	rye crackers	1 cup (150 g)	gooseberries		
	Grains*	1	grapefruit (small)		
½ cup (75g)	brown or wild rice	17-20	grapes		
½ cup (75g)	amaranth	1 cup (150 g)	guava		
½ cup (75g)	barley	1 cup (150 g)	honeydew melon		
½ cup (75g)	buckwheat	2	kiwifruit (medium)		
½ cup (75g)	non-GMO corn	6	kumquat[2]		
½ cup (75g)	kamut	free	lemons		
½ cup (75g)	millet	free	limes		
1 cup (150g)	oatmeal	1 cup (150 g)	loganberries[3]		
½ cup (75g)	quinoa	½	mango		
½ cup (75g)	rye	2	nectarines		
½ cup (75g)	spelt	1	orange (large)		
½ cup (75g)	SWG** cereal	½	papaya (large)		
½ cup (75g)	raw granola	1	peach (medium)		
	Fruits*	1	pear (medium)		
1	apple (medium)	2	persimmons		
4	apricots (small)	1 cup (150 g)	pineapple		
2 oz (56 g)	avocado	2	plums (small)		
½	banana	1	pomegranate (sm)		
1 cup (150 g)	blackberries	4	prunes (small)		
1 cup (150 g)	blueberries	2 Tbsp (30 g)	raisins		
1 cup (150 g)	boysenberries	1 cup (150 g)	raspberries		
1 cup (150 g)	cantaloupe				

* Serving sizes of grains and legumes are measured cooked, those of fruits and vegetables are measured raw

** SWG = Sprouted Whole Grain (e.g. Ezekiel 4:9 products)

Free = Use as needed for seasoning

[1] Similar to a cantaloupe

[2] similar to an orange but small like a grape

[3] cross between a blackberry and raspberry

Mixed Types: Carbohydrate Choices

Serving	Legumes*	Serving	Low-Starch Veg*	Serving	Dairy and Eggs
½ cup (75g)	adzuki beans	1	artichoke	1 cup (150 g)	salad greens[2]
½ cup (75g)	black beans	1 cup (150 g)	asparagus	1 cup (30 g)	spinach
½ cup (75g)	black-eyed beans	½ cup (75g)	bamboo shoots	½ cup (75g)	squash (winter)[4]
½ cup (75g)	fava beans	1 cup (150 g)	bok choy	½ cup (75g)	turnip
½ cup (75g)	garbanzo beans	1 cup (150 g)	broccoli	1 cup (150 g)	zucchini
½ cup (75g)	great Northern beans	1 cup (150 g)	Brussels sprouts		
½ cup (75g)	green beans	1 cup (150 g)	cabbage		
½ cup (75g)	green peas	1 cup (150 g)	cauliflower		
½ cup (75g)	lentils	1 cup (150 g)	celery		
½ cup (75g)	lima beans	1 cup (150 g)	cucumber		
½ cup (75g)	mung beans	1 cup (150 g)	daikon[1]		
½ cup (75g)	navy beans	1 cup (150 g)	eggplant		
½ cup (75g)	pink beans	1 cup (150 g)	fennel		
½ cup (75g)	pinto beans	free	garlic		
½ cup (75g)	red beans	free	ginger root		
½ cup (75g)	white beans	1 cup (150 g)	jicama		
	Dairy	1 cup (150 g)	kale		
½ cup (75g)	milk (raw)	free	lettuce[2]		
6 oz (168 g)	plain yogurt	1 cup (150 g)	mushrooms		
	High-Starch Veg*	1 cup (150 g)	okra		
1 cup (150 g)	beets	5	olives		
1 cup (150 g)	carrots	1	onion (medium)		
½ cup (75g)	Jerusalem artichoke	1 cup (150 g)	pepper (bell)		
½ cup (75g)	parsnips	free	pepper (hot)		
½ cup (75g)	potato (white)	½ cup (75g)	pumpkin		
½ cup (75g)	potato (sweet)	½ cup (75g)	radishes		
¼ cup (60g)	water chestnuts	½ cup (75g)	rutabaga[3]		

* Serving sizes of grains and legumes are measured cooked, those of fruits and vegetables are measured raw

Free = Use as needed for seasoning

[1] Japanese radish

[2] Any but iceberg

[3] Similar to a turnip

[4] Orange-fleshed squashes (e.g. acorn, butternut, and kabocha)

Fat Choices: All Metabolism Types

Serving	Fat
1 tsp	olive oil
1 tsp	fish oil
1 tsp	cod liver oil
1 tsp	flax seed oil
1 tsp	raw butter
1 oz	avocado[1]
free[2]	coconut oil
1 oz	raw cheese

Note: The fat content of fattier foods such as eggs, meats, oily fish, and nuts has been accounted for in the allotted servings and calories for each metabolism type, so no separate fat servings need to be counted for these foods.

[1] Avocado is a fruit. Protein Types also may use it as a carbohydrate choice (2 ounces).

[1] The Beyond Diet Program does not limit the amount of coconut oil that you can consume each day or account for it in the Sample Meal Plans, Done for You Meal Plans and Allowable Servings Guide. A reasonable amount would be 1–2 tsp three times per day for cooking.

*Mixed Types – Remember you are using both the Protein Type choices charts and the Carb Type choices chart for your food choices.

Ideal Food Ratios for Each Metabolism Type

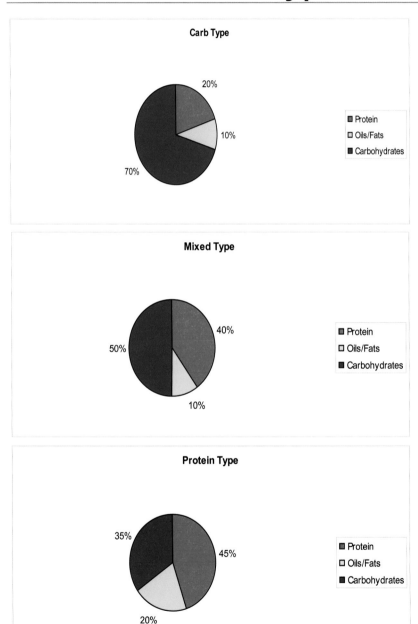

Glycemic Index Chart

	INDEX	SUGAR	DAIRY	FRUIT	GRAIN	VEGETABLES
HIGH	>100	maltose, beer, alcohol		Date		Parsnip
	90–99	glucose sports drinks			instant rice, puffed rice	
	80–89	jelly beans			Rice Chex, white rice, pretzels, Rice Krispies, Cornflakes, Rice Cakes	potato (white, baked) potato (white, instant mashed)
	70–79	Life Savers jams, jellies		watermelon	wheat cereal, graham crackers, Cheerios, bagels, whole wheat bread, white bread, millet	pumpkin rutabaga
MEDIUM	60–69	Honey		melon (all types), pineapple, raisin, banana (ripe), apricot, mango	cornmeal, rye crisp bread, shredded wheat, brown rice, brown rice pasta	Beet
	50–59			kiwifruit	corn, popcorn oatmeal, buckwheat	potato (sweet), yam, carrot, green peas

	40–49	Lactose		grape, orange	wheat bran, bulgur wheat, whole wheat pasta	beans (pinto or baked)
LOW	**30–39**		yogurt, whole, milk, butter,	apple, pear strawberry	rye	tomato soup beans (navy, lima, black, or garbanzo) peas (black-eyed or dried split)
	<30	Fructose		peach, grapefruit, plum, cherry, tomato	barley rice bran	beans (kidney or lentil), peas (dried), eggplant, summer squash, cauliflower, peanuts, green vegetables[a]

Notes: On the GI scale, high-GI foods are rapid insulin inducers and should be avoided; low-GI foods are slow insulin inducers and your best choices for weight loss.

[a] Vegetables with a GI of ~15 are ideal carbohydrate servings: artichoke, asparagus, broccoli, celery, cucumber, green bean, lettuce, green bell pepper, spinach, and zucchini.

Source: Adapted from Wolcott and Fahey 2000, 272–274.

Good, Better, Best

	Good	Better	Best!
Meat	Hormone-free, antibiotic free	Organic, hormone-free, antibiotic free	Organic free-range, grass-fed, hormone-free, antibiotic free
Dairy	Hormone-free, antibiotic free	Organic, hormone-free, antibiotic free	Raw, certified organic (or avoid altogether)
Eggs	Whole, organic eggs	Whole, organic eggs rich in Omega-3s	Whole, grass-fed, free-range eggs (from a local farm)
Bread	Whole grain breads	Spelt bread, rice bread	Sprouted Whole Grain (SWG bread)
Grains	No white/enriched grains	No wheat. Choose spelt or rye instead.	No gluten. Choose grains like quinoa, oats (make sure they're gluten free), and brown/wild rice.
Produce	Incorporate fresh fruits and vegetables into your daily meal plans.	Purchase organic fruits and vegetables from the list of produce that has been shown to have the highest levels of pesticide residue in the shopping section.	Check out your local farmers' markets for non-synthetically pesticide grown local produce. If shopping at the grocery store, purchase all organic produce.

	Good	Better	Best!
Seafood	Canned wild-caught seafood	Frozen wild-caught seafood	Fresh wild-caught seafood
Sweeteners	Truvia, Stevia products that may contain traces of maltodextrin. Xylitol: completely natural, but does have the potential to cause stomach discomfort.	Raw honey and pure maple syrup: healthy choices but should be used in moderation.	Stevia: almost free of calories, doesn't trigger a rise in blood sugar.
Alcohol	Limit alcohol consumption. A good alcohol option is vodka on the rocks; fruit juice only adds empty sugar calories. The best brand is Chopin, which is made from potatoes, not wheat.	Keep alcohol intake to 1-3 glasses per week. A better alcohol option is organic red wine. The rice flavor encourages you to drink slowly. Red wine also contains fewer calories and carbohydrates than other types of alcohol.	Cut out alcohol completely.

	Good	Better	Best!
Flours	Whole wheat flour: better choice than all-purpose flour.	Spelt flour, oat flour, millet flour.	Almond flour, coconut flour, rice flour. With the popularity of many people going "gluten free" there is no shortage of recipes you can find using these delicious flours. They are also very readily available to purchase at most supermarkets and can also be found online.
Snacks	Organic "snack foods," store-bought trail mix	Crunch Bars	Make your own! Visit the Recipes section of beyonddiet.com for ideas!

	Good	Better	Best!
Restaurants	Follow the guidelines set out in this article: http://go.beyonddiet.com/EatingOutEatingHealthy	eatwellguide.org	Keep eating out to a minimum (save it for cheat days). There are so many delicious recipes on Beyond Diet, you'll feel like you're eating out anyway!
Condiments	Organic condiments	Organic, sugar-free, store-bought condiments	Make your own! There are recipes on the site for ketchup, mustard, BBQ sauce, mayonnaise, and many more!
Beverages	Tea and organic coffee. However, you need to increase your water intake to compensate for these.	Herbal teas - No need to increase your water intake to compensate for these.	WATER! Add lemon/lime (or other fruit) and/or a little stevia to your water to give it a little more taste.
Caffeine	Zevia (soda made with stevia)	Organic coffee	Wu-Long tea, Green tea

	Good	Better	Best!
Supplements	Omega-3, greens product.	Omega-3 (derived from wild fish - call the company for details on their fish), greens product (make sure it is gluten, soy and sugar free)	Isabel's Favorite Omega-3 Supplement. Daily Energy
Dressings	Store-bought olive oil-based dressings with no added sugar (ex. Neuman's Organics)	Olive oil and vinegar	Make your own!
Exercise	Make small changes in your day that will get you to move: Take the stairs instead of the elevator. Park your car far from the entrance to any store.	Incorporate a walk/swim/bike ride into your day a couple times a week.	Work out 3-4 times a week. Include cardio and strength exercises. Use Isabel's Fast Five Exercise.

So...Just Who Is Isabel De Los Rios?

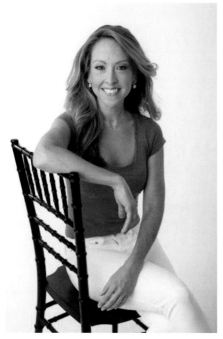

Isabel De Los Rios is a certified nutritionist and exercise specialist who has already helped more than 300,000 people all over the world lose incredible amounts of weight, regain their health and permanently change their lives. She is the author of The Beyond Diet Program and has become the #1 "go-to girl" when it comes to fat-burning nutrition by several of the most popular fitness professionals around the globe. Isabel's cutting-edge and completely different approach to nutrition is what sets her apart from all the rest. Her strategies work, hands down, as long as her simple principles are followed.

Isabel found her passion for nutrition as a teenager. The overweight daughter and granddaughter of type 2 diabetics, Isabel was told she was doomed to suffer from the same health problems as the generations who preceded her. Not willing to sit around waiting for this grim prediction to become a reality, she pored over every nutrition and diet book available in search of the answers to her family's weight and health problems. This led her to personally seek out doctors and health professionals that were using nutrition to get great results (as far as health and weight loss) with their patients and clients.

Isabel is able to educate clients and readers all over the world through her books, hundreds of online articles, seminars, and the media, focusing on the essential principles of fat-loss nutrition and achieving a healthy, toned, and vibrant body.

Isabel graduated from Rutgers University with a degree in exercise physiology (a pre-med curriculum). She is a Certified Strength and Conditioning Specialist, the highest and most advanced certification given by the National Strength and Conditioning Association. She is also a Holistic Nutrition Lifestyle Coach, certified by the Corrective Holistic Exercise Kinesiology (C.H.E.K.) Institute in San Diego, California. She counsels many special populations, including people with diabetes and heart disease, cancer survivors, and overweight individuals, as well as healthy individuals who wish to maintain their health and prevent disease.

She has since reached and maintained an ideal weight, is vibrantly healthy, and shows no indication that conditions like diabetes will affect her as they have so many in her family. She truly enjoys a high level of well-being that not only surprises most people, but motivates them to achieve what Isabel has.

REFERENCES

Batmanghelidj, F. (1992). Your Body's Many Cries for Water. Vienna, VA: Global Health Solutions, Inc.

Byrnes, Stephen (2001). The Lazy Person's Whole Foods Cookbook. Ecclesia Life Man.

Chek, Paul (2004). How to Eat, Move and Be Healthy. San Diego, CA: C.H.E.K. Institute.

Daniel, Kaayla T. (2005). *The Whole Soy Story: The Dark Side of America's Favorite Health Food.* Washington, DC: New Trends.

Fallon, Sally, with Mary G. Enig (2001). *Nourishing Traditions: The Cookbook that Challenges Politically Correct Nutrition and the Diet Dictocrats,* 2nd edition. Washington, DC: New Trends.

Fife, Bruce (2001). The Healing Miracles of Coconut Oil. Colorado Springs, CO: Health Wise.

Finger Lakes Gourmet (no date). Online recipes. www.fingerlakesgourmet.com, accessed January 2007.

Free-Gourmet-Recipes.com (no date). Healthy Recipes. www.free-gourmet-recipes.com, accessed June 2008.

Kirsch, David (2005). The Ultimate New York Body Plan. New York, NY: McGraw-Hill.

Lanctôt, Guylaine (1995). *The Medical Mafia: How to Get Out of It Alive and Take Back Our Health and Wealth.* Morgan, VT: Here's The Key Inc.

Mercola, Joseph (2005). Dr. Mercola's Total Health Program: The Proven Plan to Prevent Disease and Premature Aging, Optimize Weight, and Live Longer. Schaumburg, IL: Joseph Mercola. Available from www.mercola.com/forms/total_health_book.htm, accessed June 2008.

Mercola, Joseph (no date). *The Truth About Coconut Oil: Why It Got a Bad Rep.* articles.mercola.com/sites/articles/archive/2003/09/13/coconut-oil-part-three.aspx, accessed June 2008.

Mercola, Joseph, with Rachael Droege (2003). Trans Fat: What Exactly Is It and Why Is It So Dangerous? www.mercola.com/2003/jul/19/trans_fat.htm, accessed June 2008.

Mercola, Joseph, with Alison Rose Levy (2003). *The No-Grain Diet: Conquer Carbohydrate Addiction and Stay Slim for the Rest of Your Life.* New York, NY: Dutton. Available from www.mercola.com/nograindiet, accessed June 2008.

Quillin, Patrick (2005). Beating Cancer With Nutrition. Carlsbad, CA: Nutrition Times Press.

Regenerative Nutrition (no date). Celtic Ocean Sea Salt. www.regenerativenutrition.com/content.asp?id=30, accessed June 2008.

Rubin, Jordan S. (2004). The Maker's Diet. Lake Mary, FL: Siloam.

Sears, Al (no date). Dr. Sears Made a Mistake … Doctor House Call 78. www.alsearsmd.com/content/index.php?id=doctor_house_call_78&no_cache=1&sword_list[]=Coconut&sword_list[]=Oil, accessed June 2008.

Simopoulos, Artemis P., and Jo Robinson (1998). *The Omega Diet: The Lifesaving Nutritional Program Based on the Diet of the Island of Crete.* New York, NY: Harper Collins.

Wild Oats Marketplace (no date). *Online Recipes.* www.wildoats.com, accessed January 2007. (Editor's note: Wild Oats is now Whole Foods Market. Visit the Whole Foods Recipe Index: www.wholefoodsmarket.com/recipes/index.html, accessed June 2008.)

Wolcott, William, and Trish Fahey (2000). The Metabolic Typing Diet. New York, NY: Doubleday.